CW00506045

# Coping with Sickness

## Medicine, Law and Human Rights – Historical Perspectives

# European Association for the History of Medicine and Health Publications

Editors on behalf of the European Association for the History of Medicine and Health
*Robert Jütte and John Woodward*

## HISTORY OF MEDICINE, HEALTH AND DISEASE SERIES

1 Coping with Sickness: Historical Aspects of Health Care in a European Perspective
   *edited by John Woodward & Robert Jütte*

2 Coping with Sickness: Perspectives on Health Care, Past and Present
   *edited by John Woodward & Robert Jütte*

3 Coping with Sickness: Medicine, Law and Human Rights – Historical Perspectives
   *edited by John Woodward & Robert Jütte*

## NETWORK SERIES

1 Essays in the History of the Physiological Sciences
   *edited by Claude Debru* (Rodopi, 1995)

2 Pathology in the 19th and 20th Centuries: The Relationship between Theory and Practice
   *edited by Cay-Rüdiger Prüll*

3 Culture, Knowledge, and Healing: Historical Perspectives of
   Homeopathic Medicine in Europe and North America
   *edited by Robert Jütte, Guenter B. Risse and John Woodward*

## RESEARCH GUIDE SERIES

1 Institutes for the History of Medicine and Health in Europe: A Guide
   *edited by Robert Jütte*

2 A Guide to Archives and Records for the History of Medicine
   and Health Care in South Yorkshire and the North Midlands
   *Ian Ramage*

3 A Catalogue of Records Retained by Hospices and Related Organisations
   in the UK and the Republic of Ireland
   *Paul Lydon*

4 The History and Philosophy of Medicine and Health: Past, Present, Future
   *edited by Jan Sundin, Marie Clark Nelson and John Woodward*

## EVENING LECTURE SERIES

1 Ethics in Medicine: Historical Aspects of the Present Debate
   *Eduard Seidler*

2 Improving Health: A Challenge to European Medieval Galenism
   *Luis García-Ballester*

3 The Human Body, from Slavery to the Biomarket: An Ethical Analysis
   *Giovanni Berlinguer*

*Academic inquiries regarding the publications should be addressed to:*

John Woodward, Sheffield Centre for the History of Medicine,
University of Sheffield, Sheffield S10 2TN, United Kingdom

*or*

Robert Jütte, Institut für Geschichte der Medizin der Robert Bosch Stiftung,
Straussweg 17, D-70184 Stuttgart, Germany

HISTORY OF MEDICINE, HEALTH AND DISEASE SERIES

# Coping with Sickness

## Medicine, Law and Human Rights – Historical Perspectives

*Edited by John Woodward
and Robert Jütte*

European Association for the History of Medicine and Health Publications
*Sheffield 2000*

*Coping with Sickness: Medicine, Law and Human Rights – Historical Perspectives*
edited by John Woodward and Robert Jütte

First published in Great Britain in 2000
by European Association for the History of Medicine and Health Publications

Typeset by BBR, Sheffield, and printed in the UK by SRP Ltd, Exeter.

ISBN 0-9536522-0-3

European Association for the History of Medicine and Health Publications
Sheffield Centre for the History of Medicine
The University of Sheffield
Sheffield S10 2TN, UK

http://www.bbr-online.com/eahmh

# Contents

vii    Foreword
*John Woodward*

ix    Notes on Contributors

1    Medicine, Law and Human Rights
*John Woodward*

11    Victims and Experts: Medical Practitioners and the
Spanish Inquisition
*José Pardo-Tomás & Alvar Martínez-Vidal*

29    No Law, No Rights? Autopsy in Germany since 1800
*Cay-Rüdiger Prüll*

55    Vacher the Ripper and the Construction of the
Nineteenth-Century Sadist
*Angus McLaren*

75    Prosecution and Popularity: the Case of the Dutch Sequah, 1891–1893
*Willem de Blécourt*

91    Female Voices in Male Courtrooms – Abortion Trials in
Weimar Germany
*Cornelie Usborne*

107    'For their own good': Drug Testing in Liverpool,
West and East Africa, 1917–1938
*Helen Power*

127    Law, Medicine and Morality: A Comparative View of
Twentieth-Century Sexually Transmitted Disease Controls
*Roger Davidson & Lutz D.H. Sauerteig*

149 Defining Brain Death: The German Debate in Historical Perspective
   *Claudia Wiesemann*

171 Consolidated Bibliography

201 Index

# Foreword

THIS IS THE THIRD AND FINAL VOLUME derived from the series of conferences with the overall theme of 'Coping with Sickness' which had the co-sponsorship and financial support of the European Science Foundation and the Euroconferences Activity of the European Union. The conference, for which I took responsibility with colleagues from the Scientific Board of the European Association for the History of Medicine and Health, was held in Castelvechio di Pascoli in Italy in 1997. The European Association for the History of Medicine and Health gratefully acknowledges this core support and provision of facilities which, from 1993 to 1997, enabled the conferences to take place.

Health and welfare systems are under close scrutiny across all European states and this volume presents an historical perspective on many of the debates. It is not merely the cost of supporting various forms of welfare states which is being examined and the means of raising the necessary income, be it public taxation and/or private finance, but, in relation to this volume, the ever-expanding issues related to legislative regulation and ethical issues governing the relations between the medical profession and the lay population. Current debates range from choices concerning euthanasia to the taking of and research on body parts without or without the consent of relations. There is more scrutiny and use of regulatory authorities to ensure that improper methods and incompetent persons are removed, however, often after a revelation of impropriety or incompetence. Professional academics, be they doctors, historians, politicians or philosophers, are contributing to the legal and ethical issues as well as providing an historical and political context.

It has been an irony that I, as a co-editor of this volume, have been 'coping with sickness' throughout the gestation period. I am grateful to my co-editor and to the contributors for their patience as I prolonged the production of the volume beyond the normal expectation.

*Dr John Woodward, B.A., D.Phil.,*
*Past-President of EAHMH.*

# Notes on Contributors

ROGER DAVIDSON is Reader in Economic and Social History at the University of Edinburgh and was a Wellcome Research Fellow 1996–97. He has published widely on the social history of venereal disease in the twentieth century and on its role in the regulation of sexuality by central and local government. He is currently completing a book on *Dangerous Liaisons: The Social History of VD in Twentieth-Century Scotland* and preparing a co-edited volume on *VD and European Society since 1870*.

WILLEM DE BLÉCOURT is Associate Fellow in the History Department at Warwick University and Honorary Research Fellow at the Huizinga Institute of Cultural History, Amsterdam. He is the author of numerous publications in Dutch, English and German on witchcraft, irregular healing and popular culture. His monograph on irregular women healers in the Netherlands, 1850–1930, has just been published.

ROBERT JÜTTE is Director of the Institute for the History of Medicine of the Robert Bosch Foundation and Professor of History at the University of Stuttgart, Germany. He has published extensively on German and European urban, cultural, medical and social history. His most recent book is *Geschichte der Alternativen Medizin* (Munich, 1996). He is a member of the Scientific Board of the German Medical Association and Secretary of the European Association for the History of Medicine and Health.

ÀLVAR MARTÍNEZ-VIDAL is Lecturer in History of Medicine at the Autonomous University of Barcelona, Spain. He has studied some issues of the so-called Spanish *novator* movement, from neuroanatomical ideas to court medicine, in his books *Neurociencias y revolución científica en España* (Madrid, 1989), and *El nuevo sol de la medicina en la Ciudad de los Reyes* (Zaragoza, 1992). With María Luz López Terrada he coordinated the monographic volume devoted by the journal *Dynamis* (1996) to the Royal

Tribunal of the Protomedicato. He is currently editing, with José Pardo-Tomás, the correspondence of Juan Muñoz y Peralta (c.1665–1746), the first president of the *Regia Sociedad de Medicina* of Seville.

ANGUS MCLAREN is Professor of History at the University of Victoria, Canada and a member of the editorial board of the *Journal of the History of Sexuality*. The author of many books and articles dealing with the history of fertility control, eugenics and sexuality, his most recent studies include *The Trials of Masculinity: Policing Sexual Boundaries, 1870–1930* (University of Chicago Press, 1997), and *Twentieth-Century Sexuality: A History* (Blackwell, 1999).

JOSÉ PARDO-TOMÁS is Researcher at the Department of History of Science of the Institute "Milà i Fontanels" (CSIC, Barcelona, Spain). He has published on the history of medicine, of natural history, and of scientific books, and is the author of the monographic volumes *Ciencia y censura. La Inquisición española y los libros científicos en los siglos XVI y XVII* (Madrid, 1991), *Las primeras noticias sobre plantas americanas* (Valencia, 1993), and *La influencia de Francisco Hernández* (Valencia, 1996), among others. From 1995 he has published along with Alvar Martínez-Vidal a number of works on the diffusion of new science and modern medicine in seventeenth- and eighteenth-century Spain.

HELEN POWER is Wellcome Award Lecturer in the School of History/Department of Medicine at the University of Liverpool. Her research interests have focused on the history of tropical medicine in temperate and tropical countries, and the relationship of this discipline to other aspects of medical science and practice at national and international levels. Her first book is *Tropical Medicine in the Twentieth Century: A History of Liverpool School of Tropical Medicine* (London, 1999).

CAY-RÜDIGER PRÜLL is research assistant at the Institute for the History of Medicine at the University of Freiburg im Breisgau, Germany, where he teaches medical history. At the moment, he is working on his habilitation-thesis about the history of pathology in Berlin and London between 1900 and 1945. His doctoral thesis deals with the history of the medical faculty of the University of Giessen, Germany (1750–1918). His main research topic is the social history of modern medicine and science, in particular the history of pathology (including the history of autopsies in the 19th and 20th centuries) and psychiatry. Furthermore, he has worked on medical history museology.

LUTZ D.H. SAUERTEIG, formerly a Research Fellow at the Institute for Modern History, University of Munich, has since 1994 held the post of Lecturer and Research Fellow at the Institute for the History of Medicine, University of Freiburg, Germany. He has published on the history of sexuality and venereal disease in Germany and England. His latest publications include the monograph *Krankheit, Sexualität, Gesellschaft: Geschlechtskrankheiten und Gesundheitspolitik in Deutschland in 19. und frühen 20. Jahrhundert* (Stuttgart, Franz Steiner, 1999); 'Sex, Medicine and Morality during the First World War' (in R. Cooter & M. Harrison (eds.), *War, Medicine and Modernity, 1860–1945*, Stroud, Sutton Publishing, 1998); and 'Sexual Education in Germany from the Eighteenth to the Twentieth Centuries' (in L.A. Hall, F.X. Eder & G. Hekma (eds.), *Sexual Cultures in Europe*, vol. 2, Manchester Univeristy Press, 1999). He is currently researching the medical marketplace in twentieth-century Germany.

CORNELIE USBORNE is Reader in History at University of Surrey Roehampton London. She is the author of *The Politics of the Body in Weimar Germany. Women's reproductive rights and duties* (London and Michigan, 1992) and co-editor of *Gender & Crime in Modern Europe* (London, UCL Press, 1999). She is currently writing a monograph on *Cultures of Abortion in Weimar and Nazi Germany*. She is a member of the executive committee of the Society for the Social History of Medicine.

CLAUDIA WIESEMANN is Director of the Institute for Medical Ethics and History of Medicine at Göttingen University. Her focus of research lies on the social history of medical ethics in the twentieth century. She has published on the ethical problems of brain death definition as well as on the history of brain death. Recently she edited *Medizin und Ethik im Zeichen von Auschwitz. 50 Jahre Nürnberger Ärtzeprozeß* (together with A. Frewer) and *Die Grenzen des Anderen. Medizingeschichte aus postmoderner Perspektive* (together with T. Schnalke).

JOHN WOODWARD is Senior Lecturer in Economic and Social History in the Department of History at the University of Sheffield, United Kingdom and Co-Director of the Sheffield Centre for the History of Medicine. He has published in the social history of medicine and in historical demography, including editing with Robert Woods *Urban Disease & Mortality in Nineteenth Century England* (Batsford, 1984) and he co-edited and contributed to *Coping with Sickness. Historical Aspects of Health Care in a European Perspective* (EAHMH Publications, 1995) and *Coping with Sickness. Perspectives on Health Care, Past and Present* (EAHMH Publications, 1996).

He is a past member of the Executive Committee of the Society for the
Social History of Medicine and of the Editorial Board of *Social History of
Medicine*. Currently, he is President and a member of the Council and of the
Scientific Board of the European Association for the History of Medicine
and Health.

# Medicine, Law and Human Rights

## John Woodward

IF WE ARE TO BELIEVE two distinguished practitioners of medicine human beings have important dilemmas to reconcile when considering the title of this paper. Wilhelm von Leibnitz was quoted as commenting 'I often say a great doctor kills more people than a great general' whilst that epitome of a great doctor, William Osler, in his 'Science and Immortality' wrote 'the desire to take medicine is perhaps the greatest feature which distinguishes man from animals'.[1] Here is the very essence of the issues addressed in this volume for mankind has a yearning to preserve and to enhance health but, at the same time, there is an inherent possibility of danger in the practice of medicine, whether regular and irregular, not merely questions related to efficacy. Medicine and access to medical care has become of increasing concern in the years at the turn of the millennium as the true costs of care and the perceived needs of populations (at least in the developed world) are articulated – whilst, at the same time, those populations also perceive a maximum amount they are prepared to pay for such care – either through state-supported or voluntary insurance schemes. Thus, the end result is forms of rationing within finite allocated resources. Overlaying these issues is the role of the medical profession and the skills it proclaims to profess. In all countries members of the medical profession are criticised either for over-riding the wishes of the patient or for degrees of incompetence and, indeed, inflicting real damage (sometimes, leading to death) on the patient.

How is it that we have reached this point of very real dilemmas? On the one hand, the demands for medical care and, yet, the dissatisfaction with that care. Infinite demands and limited resources (and competence). Any conventional history of the medical profession (in whatever country) usually lists the characteristics of a profession and produces evidence from medicine which fits those characteristics. Issues related to competence and ethics are dealt with by standardised syllabuses for education and a registration system with an ethical body overseeing practice. However, more recent histories of the profession reveal a lack of homogeneity within medical practice – heterogeneity is the watchword. Be it differences between the general practitioner and the hospital consultant in Britain, the distinctions between the various specialised practitioners in the United States where general practice barely exists, to the various recognised forms of practice in Germany from the homeopath to the specialised hospital surgeon, as examples.[2] Despite regulation by law, within this spectrum of medical care, the patient finds it difficult to have his/her voice heard and, despite human rights legislation at national and international levels, is hampered in bringing actions against doctors (as, indeed, against other professionals in society). In recent years, cases of significant malpractice have been brought to the public's attention. It has been evident in Britain, for example, that the medical profession, its central regulatory authorities and local administrations have failed to take speedy action and many patients have suffered at the hands of incompetent and ethically questionable doctors (and dentists). However, the present depth of feeling may lead to a review of the professional bodies and their role in regulation. Nevertheless, the very mark of a true profession is self-regulation and governmental authorities will have to be very effective in persuading the medical profession to change the nature of reporting of incompetence and the constituent parts of the regulatory panels.

This volume examines populations, patients, doctors and other healers in their relations with each other in different time frames, different cultures and under different forms of political arrangements. The rights (or not) of the individual (which are often gender-specific) are at the very centre of these studies. Irrespective of the time or culture there are a number of common themes which link these studies and have a relevance for our current debates on rights, consent and ethics in medicine.

The paper on Spain examines the role of doctors in an inquisitorial regime which defines individuals who are outwith the bounds of the society. This is analogous to the work of Susan Solomon in the first volume of *Coping with Sickness* on the Kamlyks in post-Revolutionary Russia who were defined as the 'other'.[3] The authors, in their careful study, demonstrate that their 'exposition of some of the events involving medical practitioners implicated in this persecution will raise some questions of importance, not only with regard to the links between healers and the Inquisition, but also to the general problem of the relationship between medicine and law, especially with the social practices in which both theoretical worlds meet.'[4] They show that a significant aspect of the work of the doctors was not just '… caring for the state of health of prisoners held in Inquisitorial prisons' but was also '… providing expert evaluation with regard to specific expert evidence as well as the duty of advising and reporting back to the inquisitors on aspects relating to their particular field.'[5] In fact, having a recognised expertise, '… doctors and surgeons in the service of authority, in this specific case the Spanish Holy Office, took an active role in the mechanisms of social control and became effective collaborators with the authorities in their fight against crime (in this case, heresy and all its possible implications) and "offenders" (from the Catholic point of view, Crypto-Jews, Moriscos, Protestants, sodomites, bigamists, blasphemers, and so on).'[6]

The power of the medical profession is demonstrated by the essay by Prüll which shows that autopsy in Germany is inter-linked with the rise of morbid anatomy. However, there is also a resistance to autopsy, especially in the Weimar Republic where there was no legal regulation: 'The legal situation remained open, fostering not only expert discussions but also a dispute between pathologists and the patient's relatives.'[7] Today, the performance or not of an autopsy is an ethical issue and some pathologists and physicians suggest that the creation of an autopsy law in Germany would remove any disputes with relatives and autopsy would have a real future. Prüll argues that '… it is not at all obvious whether an increasing number of autopsies leads to better medical care of the people. On the contrary, pathologists would betray their own interests and influence as physicians by creating such a law, as there would no longer be the opportunity for individual decision-making appropriate to the respective cases.'[8] He suggests that, in the past, formal regulations inhibited the relatives in refusing an autopsy: 'Undermining someone's right to refuse an autopsy cannot be justified by referring to the advantage of autopsy for society's health care, because in doing so one would claim the right to commit an offence against individual rights, especially against the ethical principle of "informed consent".'[9] However, how can decisions be taken about the performing of an autopsy? Legislation would probably violate the interests of the medical profession and the relatives: '… pathologists and patients or relatives of patients should start to discuss autopsy on equal terms. No law, no rights? Human rights and the right to perform postmortems exist independently of any law and these rights are best preserved when every case is solved individually.'[10]

Thus, does the individual or members of the family have any rights over his/her body at the time of death? To whom does the body belong? As MacLaren suggests in his perceptive study of a sadist in '… the criminological world of the 1890s the Italian stress on biological determinism was being usurped by the French focus on pathological social forces.'[11] There was a growing understanding of the very nature of the human being and the development of the mind. A determinist view based on nature was being challenged by a view which incorporated aspects of nurture. 'If the term "sadism" was increasingly employed by public commentators at the end of the century that did not mean that there was any necessary increase in violent sexual acts nor any real growth in psychiatric knowledge. The apparent explanatory powers of sadism, it will be suggested, were more directly related to the social and cultural pressures *fin-de-siècle* France was experiencing.'[12] Here, again, is a group of professionals attempting to occupy new ground and to assist in determining a view of a form of sexual behaviour within French society.

Regulation, however, does not always provide a secure position for the medical profession as de Blecourt demonstrates. Indeed, it can do the opposite by enhancing the lay-practitioner's status from the patient's perspective. 'Laws which were meant to curtail the illegal practice of medicine turned out to promote healers by giving them free publicity, rather than by putting a stop to their trade. In the Netherlands, a country that was envied by medical associations abroad for possessing stringent medical laws, fighting "quackery" often amounted to fighting metaphorical windmills.'[13]

Usborne rightly introduces her paper by stating that 'The practice and prosecution of abortion in the early twentieth century is a central concern both for the social historian of medicine and the social historian of crime. For the former because, as a social practice, abortion touches on an essential part of women's health – reproductive choice and the problems associated with this choice – and because it was here that the medical profession fought hard to assert its influence for policy making and to gain a monopoly in regulating and treating it. For the social historian of crime abortion constitutes a challenging problem. It was, next to infanticide, which it replaced in importance in the twentieth century, the most gender-specific crime. In addition, it was one which attracted the most controversy as one of the key delicts to efforts at criminal law reform in the early twentieth century, and what was thought of its exceptionally low detection rate, largely because of the gap between official retribution and popular tolerance. Of course, men also often had a big part in abortion, both as instigators and procurers, and they were questioned by the police and in court as witnesses or charged and punished as accomplices. But women were always far more central in the event and, in the 1920s and 1930s, both as aborting women and as abortionists, particularly as lay abortionists.'[14]

The paper on drug-testing in Africa by Power is introduced by the statement that 'Research and practice may have been overlapping activities in the minds of many practitioners if, indeed, they broke up their working day in this manner. Equally, the distinctions between patient and subject were likely to be blurred, if it is assumed the practitioner consciously considered his patient cohort in this way. This is particularly the case in the testing of new drugs when manufacturers would send samples of drugs to practitioners and ask them to try the product in the normal course of treatment and provide a report. The nature of these reports was unspecified, and there was not necessarily any uniformity between different investigators who appear to have been free to experiment with methods of administration and dosage, as part of the normal therapeutic encounter.'[15]

Davidson and Sauerteig continue the theme of sexual behaviour through the debates over legislation in Britain and Germany concerning prostitution and its consequences. 'The debate over VD raised, and indeed still continues to raise, a range of fundamental and contentious issues relating to the use of legal compulsion for the purposes of disease control, and the appropriate balance within policy-making between the interests of public health and the liberty of the individual. It has also provoked extensive discussion as to the relationship of the law to morality and sexuality, and to the discriminatory features often implicit in that relationship in terms of class, gender and race.'[16]

The closely observed and nuanced analysis by Wiesemann of recent debates over the very nature of death is of great significance. By examining the German evidence she comments that 'The arguments for and against brain death are still the same as in the sixties and seventies. What has definitely changed is the belief in the natural supremacy of scientific expertise. The definition of death has become a matter of "sub-politics". Beck's categories of simple and reflexive modernisation help to explain how different social actors such as physicians, theologians, lawyers, politicians or the media dealt with the new way of treating the dead or supposed-to-be dead in different periods. The social consensus on modernisation that once allowed systematic misunderstandings of the nature of the concept of brain death to be ignored has now broken down. Whereas in simple modernity the new concept of death was considered but a minor side effect of medical progress, it has now become a risk of scientific development that has to be managed politically and is being used to regain social control over medical science.'[17]

These are all issues which, from whatever time-period, country or
culture, have a contemporary resonance. The increasing number of volumes
and articles which are being published on the boundaries of law, medicine
and society demonstrate that present society has real issues and dilemmas to
face.[18] Yet this is a recent phenomenon for, as Robert Baker has commented,
'For the best and worst of reasons, there has been little primary research on
the history of medical ethics. Among the more elevated reasons for the
paucity of scholarship are beliefs about the nature of ethics itself. The subject
is sometimes conceptualised in terms of ahistoric universal principles,
insusceptible to change, and hence lacking history – except in the realm of
interpretation. Other scholars view history from the perspective of social
science and tend to envision ethics as a mere epiphenomenon of more
fundamental socio-economic forces. These forces effectively discourage
serious historical scholarship.'[19] Yet, medical ethics over time has been
subject to elements of continuity and of change where there have been many
conflicts between humanists and technologists and by bioethics based on
human rights and patient's real choices, given full information. A review
article suggests that, in Germany, much of the recent history of medicine,
particularly of the type represented here, has been haunted by the Holocaust
but that this means that many historians find it difficult '... to disengage
themselves from this framework by stressing the autonomy and self-
rationality of the topics under investigation.'[20] The criticism of much of the
present historical study is that a number of relevant issues and approaches
remain missing: '... a patient-orientated history which investigates the
complex relationship between healer and sufferer ... This must include the
point of view not just of the doctor or non-medical practitioner and the
patient, but also of the patient's family and of all those others who play a role
in the wider healing process. Add to this feminist critiques of medicine and
anthropological approaches and we have a recipe which promises fresh
reflections on such interesting problems as medical power, the gendered
conceptions of the human body, the significance of different belief systems,
and the relationship between culture and biology.'[21] Yet, Giovanni
Berlinguer in his important study of the human body suggests that, despite
development of thought and theories of modernisation, the problems
associated with, in his case, bio-ethics, are not behind us. Equally, however,
he suggests that we should not be simplistic in just transferring knowledge
and experience from one culture and time to other cultures and times.[22] A
carefully argued example, however, of transfer can be seen in the work of
Arthur Kleinman who offers the thought that there needs to be '... an
analysis of the interaction between collective and individual, social and

subjective (levels or facets) of reality.'[23] This suggests a critique of the 'individual rights' model of bio-ethics and recommends that an over-arching view is required. As a social historian of medicine, these are of prime concerns to this author who believes that medicine cannot be divorced from its social, political and cultural context. However, what is different here from some of the previous work in the social history of medicine is that the authors in this volume are dealing with great men, with technical change and with the impact of increasing scientific knowledge on medicine and on medical practice. It was the great men who determined the role of medicine in all the periods and contexts examined in these papers be they from the early modern to the modern period. Yet, of course, it is the impact of their role on the ordinary people which comes through in these analyses. A fitting conclusion to 'medicine, law and human rights'.

## Notes

1   Sir William Osler, *Science and Immortality* (Boston, 1904), p. 2.

2   Examples of recent work would include P. Starr, *The Social Transformation of American Medicine* (New Haven, 1982); I. Waddington, *The Medical Profession in the Industrial Revolution* (Dublin, 1984), and the essays in Robert Jütte, Guenter B. Risse & John Woodward (eds.): *Culture, Knowledge and Healing: Historical Perspectives of Homeopathic Medicine in Europe and North America* (Sheffield, 1998).

3   Susan Gross Solomon, 'The Health of the Other: Medical Research and Empire in 1920s Russia' in John Woodward & Robert Jütte (eds.): *Coping with Sickness: Perspectives on Health Care, Past and Present* (Sheffield, 1996), pp. 137–160.

4   José Pardo-Tomás & Alvar Martínez-Vidal, 'Victims and Experts: Medical Practitioners and the Spanish Inquisition', this volume, p. 12.

5   Ibid., p. 13.

6   Ibid., p. 22.

7   Cay-Rüdiger Prüll, 'No Law, No Rights? Autopsy in Germany since 1800', this volume, p. 42.

8   Ibid., p. 42.

9   Ibid., p. 42.

10  Ibid., pp. 42–43.

11  Angus McLaren, 'Vacher the Ripper and the Construction of the Nineteenth-Century Sadist', this volume, p. 59.

12  Ibid., pp. 55–56.

13  Willem de Blécourt, 'Prosecution and Popularity: the Case of the Dutch Sequah, 1891–1893', this volume, p. 86.

14  Cornelie Usborne, 'Female Voices in Male Courtrooms – Abortion Trials in Weimar Germany', this volume, p. 91.

15  Helen Power, '"For their own good": Drug Testing in Liverpool, West and East Africa, 1917–1938', this volume, p. 109.

16  Roger Davidson & Lutz Sauerteig, 'Law, Medicine and Morality: A Comparative View of Twentieth-Century Sexually Transmitted Disease Controls', this volume, pp. 127–28.

17  Claudia Wiesemann, 'Defining Brain Death: The German Debate in Historical Perspective', this volume, pp. 159–60.

18  Examples of such literature would include B.J. Good, *Medicine, rationality and experience* (Cambridge, 1994); C.G. Helman, *Culture, Health and Illness* (4th ed.) (Oxford & Woburn MA, 2000) and the volumes noted by Roger Cooter in his critical review 'The Resistible Rise of Medical Ethics', *Social History of Medicine*, 8 (1995), 257–70 referred to in my 'Health Care, Past and Present' in John

Woodward & Robert Jütte (eds.), *Coping with Sickness: Perspectives on Health Care, Past and Present* (Sheffield, 1996), pp. 1–13.

19  R. Baker, 'Medical Ethics' in W.F. Bynum & R. Porter (eds.), *Companion Encyclopedia of the History of Medicine* (London & New York, 1993), Vol. 2, p. 852. This essay surveys the history of medical ethics, codification and legal regulation from Hippocrates to the present day.

20  Cornelie Usborne & Willem de Blecourt, 'Pains of the past. Recent Research in the Social History of Medicine in Germany', *Bulletin of the German Historical Institute*, 21 (1999), 6. The books reviewed are: M. Berg & G. Cocks (eds.), *Medicine and Modernity. Public Health and Medical Care in Nineteenth- and Twentieth-Century Germany*, (New York & Cambridge, 1997); U. Gerrens, *Medizinisches Ethos und theologische Ethik. Karl und Dietrich Bonhoeffer in den Auseinandersetzungen um Zwangssterilisation und 'Euthanasie' im Nationalsozialismus* (Munich, 1996); S. Stockel, *Sauglingsfursorge zwisischen sozialer Hygiene und Eugenik. Das Beispiel Berlins im Kaiserreich und in der Weimarer Republik* (Berlin & New York), 1996; C. Regin, *Selbsthilfe und Gesundsheitpolitik. Die Naturheilbewegung im Kaiserreich (1889 bis 1914)* (Stuttgart, 1995) and M. Dinges (ed.), *Medizinkritische Bewegungen im Deutschen Reich (ca. 1870–ca. 1933)*, Stuttgart, 1996.

21  Ibid., p. 20.

22  G. Berlinguer, *The Human Body. From Slavery to the Biomarket: An Ethical Analysis* (Sheffield, 1999).

23  A. Kleinman, 'Suffering in China and the West: The Challenge of an Interpersonal Locus of Experience to the Hypertrophy of Individual Autonomy in Health' in J. Woodward & R. Jutte (eds.), *Coping with Sickness...*, op. cit., p. 49.

# Victims and Experts: Medical Practitioners and the Spanish Inquisition

*José Pardo-Tomás & Alvar Martínez-Vidal*

## Introduction

THE RELATIONSHIP BETWEEN the Spanish Inquisition and medical practitioners has been considered traditionally from the same perspective – the healer as victim of the inquisitorial machine. Since the birth of inquisitorial studies in the early nineteenth century, many scholars have approached this subject from a multiplicity of angles.[1] This general tendency should not be a surprise, because throughout the more than three-century life of the Holy Office, numerous cases of physicians, surgeons, apothecaries and other healers figure prominently among the thousands of victims of its activities. There is, however, a less researched side to the relationship between the Spanish Inquisition and medical practitioners which is, nonetheless, of great interest. This is in reference to the existence of physicians and surgeons who worked for the Holy Office. At the same time, by studying the encounter of the healer with the Inquisition some issues emerge of great interest in furthering knowledge of the reality of medical practice in the society of imperial Spain, especially the connections between different medical practitioners and between them and their patients.

This study will attempt to consider all these aspects in conjunction with each other. First, a general portrayal of the figures of Holy Office medical practitioners, covering both their social status and their specific activities within the institution will be given. Secondly, a framework in which particular members of the medical profession became implicated as victims before the Inquisition will be attempted. Thirdly, an analysis of the diverse facets posed by the study of the relationship between healers and the Inquisition at a specific moment in history: that of the last great repression of the converso minority, unleashed between 1715 and 1730 and which reached its peak with the trials carried out during a five year period from 1720 to 1725, will be suggested. Finally, this exposition of some of the events involving medical practitioners implicated in this persecution will raise some questions of importance, not only with regard to the links between healers and the Inquisition, but also to the general problem of the relationship between medicine and law, especially with the social practices in which both theoretical worlds meet.

## Holy Office Physicians and Surgeons

IT IS ESSENTIAL TO RECALL that the Spanish Inquisition, first and foremost, was a court subject to an established legal, procedural and penal regulation which was common, to a large extent, to the rest of the courts operating within the political framework of the Hispanic monarchy. At the head of this court the Holy Office had a number of judges, the so-called inquisitors, who prepared trials, laid down the judicial proceedings to be followed, presided over the interrogation of, and the taking of statements from, both witnesses and the accused and, finally, passed sentences. The Inquisition, like other courts of the time, had its own prisons, where those awaiting trial were held together with people already serving prison sentences.[2]

From the time of their consolidation throughout the realms of the Hispanic crown in the mid-sixteenth century, the diverse district courts had as officers a physician and a surgeon, with their salaries, privileges and perks that came with the appointment.[3] In this sense, the Holy Office behaved like so many other European courts of law of the time requiring the presence of qualified personnel to give their expert opinion with the aim of informing their ruling. The happiness of the kingdom and the security of people depended on the tranquillity and domestic peace which the prince, according to Renaissance writers, was obliged to provide for his states. Giving the appropiate punishment to those who broke the law, disturbed social harmony and instigated discord, served to guarantee the honour and estates of his subjects, and to prevent disturbances and uprisings against authority. The university-educated doctor, as an expert and the possessor of officially recognised expertise, was able to aid the courts in the settlement of criminal lawsuits by giving his judgement as to whether particular acts could be considered infringements of the law and, therefore, were punishable or not. Thus, the doctor, in the service of authority, took an active role in the mechanisms of social control and became an effective collaborator with the ruler in his fight against crime and offenders.[4]

Apart from the legal traditions, canonic and civil, which linked medical practitioners with courts of law from the Late Middle Ages,[5] a series of medical texts published during the sixteenth century, classifiable under the heading of legal medicine, brought within a body of doctrine all those questions which might help physicians and surgeons carry out their duties as medical experts in trials. Monographs, such as those by Cardano and Mercurialis on poisonings, by Paré on embalmments, and Sylvaticus on simulation, as well as the compendium entitled *Methodus dandi relationes* by Ingrassia, are the most renowned. The year 1621 saw the appearance of the first systematic treatise on legal medicine: the *Quaestiones medico legales* by the papal archiatra Paolo Zacchia, which enjoyed immense influence during the seventeenth and eighteenth centuries. As well as being qualified in medicine and law, Zacchia could count on the experience he had gained as a medical expert during several decades at the Rota, the Roman court.[6]

The responsibilities of a medical practitioner serving in an Inquisitorial court covered two broad areas. First, caring for the state of health of prisoners held in Inquisitorial prisons, and secondly, providing expert evaluation with regard to specific expert evidence as well as the duty of advising and reporting back to the inquisitors on aspects relating to their particular field. Before these aspects are discussed, however, answers need to be found for such questions as: How many posts were there? What was their nature? and, What was the social status of those who filled them? The number of medical practitioners on inquisitorial tribunals was not subject to any specific regulation but followed the general trend of the number of officers serving the Holy Office, that is an almost continuous increase.[7] In fact, as far as the data reveal and taking into account local variations, at first there was seldom more than one post open to a physician and another to a surgeon in each district court but, over time, two or even three posts for each of them were not unusual. It is also true that, on occasion, such posts fell vacant for indefinite periods.[8] As with the rest of the personnel, the post of physician, surgeon or barber to an inquisitorial tribunal was for life, and was subject to the same abuses generated by practically all the public offices of imperial Castile: *de facto* hereditary transfer of ownership, sale of office, inheritance of office, transfer of ownership in life, absentee ownership, temporary surrender of ownership, etc. As for salary levels, all the data indicate that both the physician and the surgeon were among the low-earning group of officials. Their pay was comparable only with that of defence lawyers, a fact which is not unentirely symptomatic.[9] However, the salary did not exclude other sources of income, just as it did not prevent them enjoying a series of fringe benefits. On the one hand, medical costs were paid for out of the funds which had been raised by the confiscation of the prisoner's property, a measure generally taken at the very moment the individual was arrested. In this way, whenever a physician prescribed bleeding, foot-bathing, or a particular anointment, he was paid with the prisoner's property, as was the surgeon responsible for the application of these remedies, or the apothecary who prepared the medicine to be administered.[10] In other words, prisoners paid medical practitioners for any special health care. On the other hand, the Holy Office medical practitioner attended the rest of the court officials, including the inquisitors, as well as the so-called *familiares* of the Holy Office, a group of around forty or fifty direct collaborators, who acted as a police force in the service of the Inquisition. Therefore, the post was an attractive proposition for the practitioner, not so much because of the accompanying salary, but because it gave him the opportunity to build up a numerous, and above all, influential clientele.

As for social status, there can be no doubt that, as well as a regular income, the post of Inquisition medical practitioner carried with it other advantages not to be scorned at in a society where privilege and honour were the highest social values. Firstly, the medical practitioner obtained the privileges associated with the special position that an official of the Holy Office occupied in society. This took the form of the legal security provided by the exclusive jurisdiction that the Holy Office had over its officers. Secondly, the post offered also another kind of security, as the mere fact of being a member of the Holy Office implied having successfully passed an investigation into the purity of blood. This was of great utility in a society in which slur campaigns, regarding the Hebrew or Muslim origins of some of the more unprotected of its members were rife. In other words, it was much more difficult to slander the purity of lineage of somebody in the pay of the Inquisition[11].

As a result, the post of Holy Office practitioner was very appealing, and explains why such posts were so sought after. The selection of different candidates initially fell to the district inquisitors, though the final appointment was made by the Supreme Council. The fundamental criterion when it came to choosing a medical practitioner for the court, once the necessary purity of blood investigation had been overcome, was the candidate's professional reputation. In many cases, he would already have become a *familiar* of the Inquisition.[12] Indeed, in this aspect, there was an interchange of honours between the two parties. The Inquisition gave social respectability and legal privileges to its physician; in return, given the latter's professional reputation, it received further social legitimacy for its activities. This legitimacy was derived from the very prestige of university-based medicine, the art of healing rooted in the academic training of those who practised it and, ultimately, in the authority, sanctioned by religious orthodoxy, of an intellectual tradition which went back to the works of Hippocrates and Galen. Therefore, it is hardly surprising to find that the court physicians of Valencia, Barcelona, Zaragoza, Seville, Valladolid or Granada (all being university cities) were appointed typically from among the professors of the medical faculty.[13] As for the prestige acquired by the doctor, it is sufficient to say that in over fifty cases of printed medical works from the sixteenth and seventeenth centuries, the authors make reference on the title page to being Holy Office physicians or *familiares*.[14]

The specific question of what the Inquisition's medical practitioners actually did in practice now needs consideration, taking note of the twofold nature of their responsibilities: the medical care for prisoners and the expert evaluation and reports for inquisitors. The main burden of monitoring a prisoner's health fell on the surgeon, and, if there was one available to the court, on the barber. It was their duty to shave prisoners and to attend to specific necessities as they arose or as the physician ordered. The physician himself did not usually visit patients on a regular basis, but only when summoned by the prison governor, after consultation with the inquisitors, whether it be to certify the death of a prisoner in the cells, or for cases of requests for hospitalisation or certain cases of pregnancy amongst female prisoners.[15] Providing expert evaluation might entail supplying medical evidence in the form of reports on a different sort of matter, requested by the inquisitors. Although written legal procedure with regard to these functions is not abundant the court transcripts kept in the inquisitorial archives allow a varied casuistry of medical expertise to be established. Without any doubt, the inquisitors required most often a physician's report in cases where torture was involved. Unfortunately for those who suffered it, torture was standard procedural practice in the courts of all *ancien régime* societies. This means that the use of torture was integral to penal procedure and was applied at the judge's discretion, whenever he felt it necessary to obtain evidence which would prove the prisoner's guilt or innocence.[16] In this respect, the Inquisition used torture like any other court and, in general, despite what is commonly believed, in a less frequent and less cruel manner.[17] The cruelty of inquisitorial torture lay not so much in the physical side, but in the intention behind it. Given that the offences which were of concern to the Holy Office were essentially of a spiritual nature, the use of torture was designed always to obtain the prisoner's admission of guilt, with the irrational idea that only in this way could their soul be saved from eternal damnation: a greater resistance to pain did not prove the sinner's innocence, but rather his or her stubbornness. It is this aspect which makes inquisitorial torture so despicable. The physician's role in the practice of torture was to make a preliminary examination of the prisoner, and to determine if he or she was in a fit state to withstand torture or if there was any impediment to a particular torture being used. There is no clear evidence to suggest that medical evaluation helped either to restrict or facilitate the work of the torturer.[18] The casuistry was very varied and, rather than obeying a clearly laid down code of ethics, physicians' decisions seem to have been spontaneous in nature. Faced with the infinite variety of cases and the infinite variety of responses from the inquisitorial physician, the existence of a code of conduct which encompassed anything, including indifference and cruelty, can only be affirmed. Another type of medical report requested with relative frequency by the inquisitor is not related to trial procedure but to the establishment of particular punishments at the time of passing sentence. Among the range of penalties given by the Holy Office were those which involved corporal punishment, especially the lash. In these cases, the physician was asked to examine the convicted person to see if their health would stand the punishment.[19]

As for supplying medical evidence, the medical practitioners' responsibilities were logically much more varied, given the diversity of offences being tried and the multiplicity of circumstances which might require the practitioner's participation in the securing of evidence. Two groups of cases are most commonly found. First, medical opinion was necessary to validate or refute allegations, principally made by the defence, about the mental health of the accused. The physician was required by the inquisitor to inform him whether or not the prisoner was sound in mind and, therefore, conscious of having sinned, or if he or she could be exonerated on the grounds of temporary or permanent diminished responsibility. This type of allegation would be made in cases involving charges of blasphemy, diverse heretical propositions or offences of a similar nature.[20] In contrast, it does not seem that medical evaluation was often called for in cases of witchcraft or sorcery. It would appear that, in line with the mentality of the time and in agreement with the theological thinking behind inquisitorial practices, theologians took sole responsibility for these cases, leaving very little room for the opinion of a physician in a witchcraft trial. [21]

The second significant group of cases was the numerous interventions in the trials of those accused of Crypto-Judaism. One of the most important pieces of medical evidence consisted of establishing whether or not a prisoner had been circumcised. This made necessary an examination of the accused by a Holy Office surgeon, normally in the presence of the physician, who then informed the inquisitor of their findings.[22] The presentation of such damning evidence proved conclusive for the prosecution's case. It is, therefore, not surprising that this is one of the few aspects of the provision of expert evaluation about which it is possible to find explicit documented references to some sort of code of practice. In 1635, at least, and again in 1662, the Supreme Council reminded all the district courts of the usefulness and covenience of ordering the securing of this particular evidence in cases of suspected Crypto-Judaism. [23]

However, this was not all. With regard to eating habits, it was sometimes necessary to establish if the prisoner's allegation was acceptable to medical science. An example taken from a trial will illustrate this point. In the Holy Office of Toledo in 1607, a Bachelor of Medicine called Felipe de Nájera was put on trial, accused of being a Judaiser. Among the practices attributed to him by informers was apparently that of not eating pork. On being interrogated, Felipe de Nájera alleged that he had once suffered from gout and that this type of food was not good for somebody with this condition. As a Bachelor of Medicine, he had his own knowledge and the weight of authority on his side: his decision was in line with Galen's *De alimentorum facultatibus*. In the face of the prisoner's allegation, the Toledo Inquisition consulted their own physician, Doctor Gaspar López, who corroborated Nájera's opinion and the citation from Galen which he had cited.[24] The importance of this incident is not limited to its illustration of a case in which the provision of expert evidence by an Inquisition doctor was central to the establishment of proof of the offence of Judaism. Here are two physicians, face to face, on opposing sides of the issue: one as the accused, the other as the prosecution expert. Both speak the same language, both appeal to the same unquestionable authority, but each plays a completely different role. As in Nájera's case, physicians and surgeons often found themselves face to face with fellow medical practitioners, who were on the other side, in the role of victim.

## The Medical Practitioner as Victim of the Inquisition

THE SPANISH INQUISITION emerged in the latter part of the fifteenth century as a new institution, different in many aspects from the medieval Inquisition which was, by that time, practically inactive. One new

aspect of the revamped Spanish Inquisition which stands out from the rest
was its close links with royal power, and its special devotion to the repression
of the two existing religious minorities in Hispanic society: the Moriscos and
the Jewish Conversos.

For a monarchy whose interests went hand in hand with those of the
Church with regard to both domestic order and the development of a foreign
policy with an eye to expansion on the international front, the presence
of a Muslim minority at home was no longer tolerable. The obligatory
conversions decreed first in Andalusia and Castile in 1496, and some decades
later in 1526 in the territories of the Aragon crown, were the real cause of
the Morisco problem, as this minority was forced to adopt in name the
Christian religion if it wanted to survive in its own country. The Inquisition
was the instrument for imparting a 'pedagogy of fear'[25] to these new
Christians who had had baptism thrust upon them, suppressing the
continuity of Islamic practices in the heart of Morisco communities. Its
failure in this respect was total, and led, in 1609, to the expulsion of nearly
three hundred thousand Moriscos from the territories of the Catholic king.[26]
The Inquisition played an important part in the disintegration of Morisco
communities, handing out fines, introducing special taxes, and consciously
contributing to their impoverishment.

The case of the Conversos was similar, though not identical. The
significant differences between the two minorities, with regard to their
geographical distribution as well as their social integration or their economic
activities, gave rise to different responses to repression. The choice between
expulsion or obligatory conversion was put to Hispanic Jews some years
before Muslims, in 1492 in Castile and Aragon. In Portugal, the option of
exile did not exist, making the situation more dramatic there.[27] From this
moment, the Converso problem, which existed already with those groups
converted as a result of the different pogroms started a century earlier, took
on much greater proportions. A terrible period of repression began, which
the Inquisition carried out with relentless ferocity, at least until the 1520s.
Later on, the Inquisition would turn its attention sporadically to the
Judaisers, before the arrival of the last great wave of trials which took place
in the first three decades of the eighteenth century.[28] It is within this general
framework that we can place the great majority of physicians, surgeons and
healers in general who were put on trial by the Holy Office during the first
two hundred and fifty years of its existence. In fact, the Converso physician
and the Morisco healer are two prototypical inquisitorial victims.[29]
Alongside the quantitative and qualitative importance of these groups, the
few trials against Old Christian medical practitioners were isolated cases and,

without doubt, of little significance. The confrontation between Inquisition and Morisco healers was seen in terms of a struggle between academic medicine and popular forms of medical practice, steeped in magic and quackery. For the inquisitors, any inexplicable healing carried out by the Morisco practitioner could be interpreted, in principle, as having resulted from a pact with the Devil, and was therefore suspicious, especially if accompanied by strange rituals or incomprehensible invocations. With these assumptions, the Inquisition sought to undermine the Morisco communities' medical system, by attacking the medical doctrines of their healers and hindering the relationship between practitioner and patient, especially if the latter was a Christian. They were given heavy fines which came with lifetime bans on practising medicine.[30]

The Conversos did not form a community separated from the rest of Christian society. They did not have their own form of medicine, or a distinctive system of medical care. As opposed to the Moriscos, Converso physicians were fully integrated into the medical 'establishment'. As long as their Jewish origins went undiscovered, they studied at university and practised the orthodox medicine accepted by the Christian majority. In fact, though tried by inquisitorial tribunals, they were not accused of medical practice deviating from what was considered 'normal' neo-Scholastic Galenism such as spells, charms, witchcraft and so on, but for being Judaisers. In other words, for observing Jewish practices in secret, something looked upon as heresy. In order to avoid falling victim to inquisitorial persecution, many of them chose exile, others fled to the New World, whilst in the last instance, others opted for conversion, thus abandoning the religion of their ancestors. [31] In the inquisitors' eyes it was dangerous that a Converso physician, who secretely kept his faith and observed Jewish practices, should attend a Christian patient, as a patient's access to the sacraments might be jeopardised if the attending physician failed to fulfill the religious precept of inducing and encouraging confession.[32] The Converso physician thus became an easy target for rival practitioners as well as dissatisfied patients. Denouncement, something which the Holy Office constantly encouraged, was a handy weapon, easy to use and of devastating consequences for those who fell victim to the infamy.[33] Not surprisingly, the inquisitorial trials of Converso practitioners reveal a maze of rivalries between physicians, or between physicians and surgeons, or conflicts between practitioners and patients, which end up being settled in such a peculiar court.[34]

## Medical Practitioners and Inquisition in the Last Great Persecution of Conversos

AROUND 1720 THE INQUISITION seemed to have stirred itself from a period of a certain paralysis, caused by the recent military conflicts of the War of the Spanish Succession, by its own particular problems, and by relations with different sectors of power, especially the clique that had formed around the monarch.[35] This change of attitude is symbolised by the appointment to the post of Inquisitor General in July 1720 of Juan de Camargo, a man who had devoted virtually his whole career to the inquisitorial apparatus. Until his death in 1733,[36] the Inquisition was to enjoy what was, perhaps, its last flurry of activity, though it would live on for another century. The situation had, however, shown signs of changing some years before, at least as far as renewed measures of repression were concerned. These were aimed at the various families descended from Portuguese Conversos, who lived all over the Iberian peninsula and formed an especially significant group in the very capital of the kingdom, Madrid. In fact, in around 1716, trials involving members of these families began to take place not only in Madrid, but also in Toledo, Granada, and Seville. Four years later, the situation had taken on the proportions of systematic persecution, in which trials would set off a chain of further trials affecting virtually everywhere. Towards 1730, when the rate of trials and convictions seemed to be diminishing, the toll left no room for doubt. Two pieces of data reveal, first, that the number of convicted prisoners was over 2,000, with more than 200 death sentences carried out and, second, that nearly 80% of the total number of convictions, and nearly 100% of the death sentences, were for Judaism.[37]

An exact calculation of the medical practitioners convicted during the persecution from 1715 to 1730 is rather more difficult. A rough indication may be gained from an analysis of official records of sentences handed out to 1,091 prisoners in 66 *autos-da-fé*, held in different places, from 7 April 1720 to 16 December 1725, that is to say, during the peak years of the persecution. A total of 27 physicians, five barbers, three surgeons, and five apothecaries, plus one medical student, a druggist, and two doctors' widows, were condemned, all of them for being Judaisers.[38] Among the different groups of Crypto-Jewish families, that of Madrid stands out for its size, as well as for the status of some of its members. Here, a clandestine synagogue was founded in around 1707, and a rabbi appointed in about 1714. Among the dozens of testimonies and denouncements of people tried for belonging to this group of Madrid Judaisers, the names of several medical practitioners are found.[39] At least three of them were formally charged and arrested in their homes, in the early hours of 1 March 1721: the doctors Francisco de la Cruz, Juan Muñoz y Peralta and Diego Mateo Zapata.

The last two were distinguished figures in Spanish medical circles of the time, as their names were identified with the so-called 'novator' movement, started in the last years of the seventeenth century and continued in the early decades of the following one.[40] Peralta and Zapata were both founder members of the scientific 'Veneranda Tertulia' established in Seville in 1697 and officially recognised as a 'Regia Sociedad de Medicina y otras Ciencias' in 1700. Peralta was its first president, a post in which he was succeeded by Zapata. Also, in the years prior to their arrest, they had published various medical works of a markedly renovative nature, and had been drawn into the bitter controversies which raged between these 'novator' physicians and representatives of the most intransigent galenist traditionalism.[41] Despite the galenists' positions of strength and the virulence of their attacks, both Peralta and Zapata managed to raise powerful support. In fact, Peralta was made an honorary royal physician in 1700, and on his arrest in 1721 was already a fully fledged royal physician. Zapata, meanwhile, was physician to the Duke of Medinaceli as he already had been to other important court figures, including Cardinals Borja and Portocarrero. The third of the doctors arrested in Madrid in 1721, Francisco de la Cruz, had also reached prominent court status as royal family physician.[42] These three doctors' lofty social position did not save them from inquisitorial persecution, and in the case of Dr Cruz not even from a tragic ending: he died in the Inquistion cells before seeing the end of his trial, which ran its course after his death and concluded in his being burnt in effigy and his bones being exhumed and thrown on the fire. His two colleagues met a different fate. Muñoz y Peralta was released, but after a trial lasting nearly three years; Zapata was sentenced in 1725 to a year in prison and banished for ten years from the royal court, as well as having half of his wordly possessions confiscated. In this case, it seems that the Duke of Medicinaceli's protection had served at least to shorten the length of the banishment.

## Conclusions

THE TRIALS OF CRYPTO-JEWS raise many varied questions, to which it is still too soon to get satisfactory answers. In the numerous trials, the complex web of denouncements, the interrogations of witnesses, the expert evidence and reports of surgeons or physicians, and the statements of those implicated, reveal not only a tapestry of characters, but also a network of relationships between medical practitioners of varying levels, and between them and their patients. But the trials also throw up a wide range of connections with wider implications: the struggle between tradition and renovation in Spanish medicine of the era, the participation of a Jewish Converso element on the side of renovation, the underlying ideological and social motives behind inquisitorial persecution, etc. As experts, doctors and surgeons in the service of authority, in this specific case the Spanish Holy Office, took an active role in the mechanisms of social control and became effective collaborators with the authorities in their fight against crime (in this case, heresy and all its possible implications) and 'offenders' (from the Catholic point of view, Crypto-Jews, Moriscos, Protestants, sodomites, bigamists, blasphemers, and so on).

It should be stressed that the presence of medical practitioners in the Spanish inquisitorial tribunals became more and more structural than occasional. The number and functions of medical practitioners on inquisitorial boards showed a trend of almost continuous increase, involving even two or three permanent posts, with salary and benefits, for each of the fifteen local courts. A comparative perspective in the European context might reveal this to be an unusual if not peculiar feature. However, research to date lacks a satisfactory number of specific studies to establish this comparison.[43] With regard to ethical issues, it does not appear that medical expertise helped to restrict the cruelty of the judicial procedures. In fact, the practitioners' attitudes in court ranged from indifference to inhumanity, and there is no evidence of criticism of the aims and methods of the Holy Office from the medical establishment. Moreover, to be a physician or surgeon of the Inquisition gave social respectability and legal privileges; in return, the prestige of university-based medicine reinforced the social legitimacy of the activities of this tribunal. In the future it may be possible to provide satisfactory answers to some of the many questions that this research raises. The particular aim in this study has been to present a wider perspective framework than that which has traditionally been offered for this specific case. Persecuted for being Crypto-Jews or recruited as experts, victims or collaborators, Spanish medical practitioners could not avoid the obvious presence of the Holy Office in the society in which they lived.

*This article has been accomplished within the funds of the Research Project PB96-0761-C03-02 of the DGES Spanish Ministery of Education. We wish to thank Phil Grayston for his help with the English version.*

# Notes

1   An essential starting point to an understanding of early inquisitorial historiography are the works of Juan A. Llorente, *Histoire critique de l'Inquisition d'Espagne*, 4 vols (Paris, 1817–1818) and Henry C. Lea, *A History of the Inquisition of Spain*, 4 vols (New York, 1906–1907). It is impossible here to provide a complete bibliography of subsequent work on the Spanish Inquisition; up to the 1980s, the repertory of such studies totalled nearly five thousand: E. Van der Vekene, *Bibliotheca Bibliographica Historia Sanctae Inquisitionis*, 2 vols (Vacluz, 1982). As for inquisitorial studies of recent years, see the excellent overview offered by Ricardo García Cárcel, 'Ascens i decadència de la historiografia de la Inquisició', *L'Avenç*, No. 210 (January 1997), pp. 18–23. English speakers may consult two collective works of highly varied contributions: Gustav Henningsen, John Tedeschi & Charles Amiel (eds.), *The Inquisition in Early Modern Europe: Studies in Sources and Method* (Dekalb, Ill. 1984) and Angel Alcalá (ed.), *The Spanish Inquisition and inquisitorial mind* (Boulder, 1987).

2   Francisco Tomás y Valiente, 'Relaciones de la Inquisición con el aparato institucional del Estado' in Joaquín Pérez Villanueva (ed.), *La Inquisición española. Nueva visión, nuevos horizontes* (Madrid, 1980), pp. 41–60; Juan Meseguer, 'Las primeras estructuras del Santo Oficio' in *Historia de la Inquisición en España y América* (Madrid, 1984), vol. 1, pp. 370–405.

3   Lea, *A History of the Inquisition of Spain*, vol. II, pp. 248–49.

4   Guido Ruggiero, 'The Cooperation of Physicians and the State in the Control of Violence in Renaissance Venice', *Journal of the History of Medicine and Allied Sciences, 33*, 156–166 and his *Violence in Early Renaissance Venice* (New Brunswick, 1980).

5   Luis García Ballester, 'Medical Ethics in Transition in the Latin Medicine of the Thirteenth and Fourteenth Centuries: New Perspectives on the Physician–Patient Relationship and the Doctor's fee' in A. Wear, J. Geyer-Kordesch & R. French (eds.), *Doctors and Ethics: The Earlier Historical Setting of Professional Ethics* (Amsterdam & Atlanta, 1993), pp. 38–71 and his 'Ethical problems in the relationship between doctors and patients in fourteenth-century Spain: on Christian and Jewish practitioners' in Samuel S. Kottek & Luis García Ballester (eds.), *Medicine and Medical Ethics in Medieval and Early Modern Spain* (Jerusalem, 1996), pp. 11–32.

6   E.H. Ackerknecht, 'Legal Medicine in Transition (16th–18th Centuries)', *The Ciba Symposia*, 9 (1950–51), pp. 1286–1304.

7   Ricardo Garcia Cárcel, 'El funcionamiento estructural de la Inquisición inicial' in *Historia de la Inquisición en España y América*, vol. 1, pp. 405–433.

8   A complete picture of the situation in the first half of the eighteenth century can be seen in Lea, *A History of the Inquisition of Spain*, vol. 2, p. 597.

9 Lea, *A History of the Inquisition of Spain*, vol. 2, pp. 208–23; Jaime Contreras, 'Las modificaciones estructurales. Los cambios en la Península' in *Historia de la Inquisición en España y América*, vol. 1, pp. 1156–77. With regard to salaries, see the figures for the court in Madrid in 1726, offered by Juan Blázquez, *Madrid. Judíos, herejes y brujas. El tribunal de Corte, 1650–1820* (Toledo, 1990), pp. 21–22

10 Madrid, Archivo Histórico Nacional, Inquisición [from here referred to as AHN, Inquisición], lib. 632.

11 Lea, *A History of the Inquisition of Spain*, vol. 2, pp. 285–312. For purity of blood *estatutos*, Albert Sicroff's study remains indispensable: *Les controverses des status de "pureté de sang" en Espagne du XVe au XVIIe siècles* (Paris, 1960).

12 We base ourselves on various appointments taken from AHN, Inquisición, lib. 360 & 361. Elsewhere, we have studied the particular case of sixteenth-century Valencia, which constitutes a highly representative example: José Pardo-Tomás, 'Llorenç Coçar y la Inquisición valenciana' in *Homenatge al Doctor Sebastià Garcia Martínez* (Valencia, 1988), vol. 1, pp. 363–73.

13 For example, in Valencia in the sixteenth century, the university professors Lluís Collado, Llorenç Coçar, Joan Plaça, Josep Reguart, and Pasqual Rubio: Pardo Tomás, 'Llorenç Coçar y la Inquisición valenciana', pp. 367–68. In seventeenth-century Valladolid, the same was true of, amongst others, Gaspar Bravo de Sobremonte and Cipriano de Maroja Latorre; in Zaragoza, many such cases included those of Jerónimo Uguet, Jerónimo Garcés, and Bartolomé Sanahuja.

14 These data have emerged from our consultation of covers, dedications, and first drafts of a large part of printed medical output, based on that collected in José Mª. López Piñero et al., *Bibliographia Medica Hispanica*, vols. 1 (1475–1600) & 2 (1601–1700) (Valencia, 1987–1989). In addition to those cited in the preceding note, we may mention here some further examples: Bernardino de Laredo, Melchor de Villena, Nicolás Vargas Valenzuela, Juan de Figueroa, Pedro García Carrero, Alonso de Freilas, etc.

15 To mention but a few well-known examples, note the case of Juan de Valdés, imprisoned in Valladolid in 1641, already related by Lea, *A History of the Inquisition of Spain*, vol. 2, p. 523. For problems concerning pregnancy amongst female prisoners, see the case of María de Tudela, held prisoner in Madrid in 1718, cited by Julio Caro Baroja, *Los Judíos en la España Moderna y Contemporánea* (Madrid, 1986), vol. 3, p. 56ff.

16 Francisco Tomás y Valiente, 'El proceso penal', *Historia 16. Extra I* (December 1976), pp. 19–35. A general framework for torture in *ancien régime* criminal law in Francisco Tomás y Valiente, *La tortura en España. Estudios históricos* (Barcelona, 1973).

17 The idea of a lesser degree of physical cruelty in inquisitorial torture had already been put forward by Lea, *A History of the Inquisition of Spain*, vol. 3, pp. 1–3, although the same author relates a good number of cases in which this supposed milder torture is not at all apparent: Ibid., pp. 22–26.

18  To the contradictory cases related by Lea, A History of the Inquisition of Spain, vol. 3, pp. 1–35, many others may be added. It is particularly shocking, for example, to see the clearly collaborationist attitude of the doctors in response to inquisitorial torture in the case of the weaver, Alonso de Alarcón: one of them informed the inquisitors that applying torture to the prisoner's left side was pointless, as the poor craftsman had no feeling in this part of his body owing to a stroke, and therefore suggested that they should concentrate their efforts on his right side, where the rack would cause him pain; related in Tomás y Valiente, 'El proceso penal', p. 26.

19  In 1725, the doctor Diego Mateo Zapata was sentenced, amongst other punishments, to two hundred lashes. He was examined beforehand by the physician of the Cuenca court, in order to determine whether or not he would stand up to the punishment: Cuenca, Archivo Diocesano, Inquisición [from here referred to as: ADC, Inquisición], leg. 573, exp. 7065, ff. 320r–323v.

20  There are many cases of this, of which we shall give just two significant examples. Firstly, the aforementioned case of the weaver, Alonso de Alarcón, in which the inquisitors insisted on the expert testimony of at least two physicians in response to the defence's allegation of mental disorder: Tomás y Valiente, 'El proceso penal', pp. 25–26. Another case, which, moreover, affected a physician as a patient, is that of the Valencian Josep Pérez, in 1613, narrated by William Monter, Frontiers of heresy. The Spanish Inquisition from Basque Lands to Sicily (Cambridge, 1990), p. 295.

21  Gustav Henningsen, The Witches' advocate: basque witchcraft and the Spanish Inquisition, 1609–1614 (Reno, 1980).

22  Among the many cases of expert evidence on the question of circumcision, of special significance is that of the physician Diego Mateo Zapata, in ADC, Inquisición, leg. 557, exp. 6955, ff. 3v y 30r. Two very similar cases are mentioned by Caro Baroja, Los judíos, vol. 2, p. 222; and Rafael de Lera, 'La última gran persecución contra el judaísmo. El tribunal de Cuenca, 1718–1725', in J.A. Escudero, Perfiles jurídicos de la Inquisición española (Madrid, 1989), pp. 805–37.

23  Madrid, Biblioteca Nacional [from here referred to as: BNM], Ms-854, p. 60 documents a letter, agreed by the Council of the Inquisition, the so-called Suprema, to all the inquisitorial courts, dated 31 January 1635, which lays down that surgeons should examine the male prisioners testificados de judaismo, to see if they had been circumcised. In 1662, inquisitorial surgeons were reminded in similar terms of this duty.

24  AHN, Inquisición, leg. 168, exp. 1, contains the case of the bachelor Nájera, which serves to illustrate a clear case of the consequences of tension between the medical practitioner and his clientele. Brought to light by Caro Baroja, Los judíos, vol. 2, pp. 211–20; also analysed by Luis García Ballester, 'The Inquisition and minority medical practitioners in Counter-Reformation Spain', in O.P. Grell & A. Cunningham (eds.), Medicine and the Reformation (London, & New York, 1993), pp. 156–91; 176–85.

25  Bartolomé Bennassar, *L'Inquisition espagnole. XVe–XIXe siècle* (Paris, 1979), pp. 105–41.

26  The bibliography on Hispanic Moriscos is relatively abundant. An excellent synthesis, made by two of the leading specialists in the field, is that of Antonio Domínguez Ortiz & Bernard Vincent, *Historia de los moriscos. Vida y tragedia de una minoría* (Madrid, 1985). For those readers restricted to reading in English, note that Henry Charles Lea himself published the work, *The Moriscos of Spain. The Conversion and Expulsion* (London, 1901).

27  Y. Yerushalmi, *From Spanish Court to Italian Ghetto: Isaac Cardoso. A Study in Seventeenth-Century Marranism and Jewish Apologetics* (New York, 1971), pp. 21–42.

28  Jean Pierre Dedieu, 'Le quatre temps de l'Inquisition' in B. Bennassar et al., *L'Inquisition espagnole XVe–XIXe siècle* (Paris, 1979), pp. 16–41; Gustav Henningsen, 'El banco de datos del Santo Oficio. Las relaciones de causas de la Inquisición española (1550–1700)', *Boletín de la Real Academia de la Historia*, 174 (1977), pp. 547–70.

29  Luis García Ballester, 'Minorities and Medicine in Sixteenth-Century Spain: Judaizers, "Moriscos" and the Inquisition' in Samuel S. Kottek & Luis García Ballester (eds.), *Medicine and Medical Ethics in Medieval and Early Modern Spain* (Jerusalem, 1996), pp. 119–35.

30  Luis García Ballester, 'The minority of Morisco Physicians in the Spain of the 16th Century and their Conflicts in a Dominant Christian Society', *Sudhoffs Archiv*, 60 (1976), pp. 209–34; by the same author, *Los moriscos y la medicina* (Barcelona, 1984); and 'Academicism versus empiricism in practical medicine in sixteenth-century Spain with regard to Morisco practitioners' in A. Wear, R.K. French & I.M. Lonie (eds.), *The medical renaissance of the sixteenth century* (Cambridge, 1985), pp. 246–70.

31  An excellent summary of the question in the collective work: Henry Méchoulan (ed.), *Les juifs d'Espagne. Histoire d'une diaspora, 1492–1992* (Paris, 1992). Consultation should be made of the controversial but indispensable book by B. Netanyahu, *The Marranos of Spain Late 14th to Early 16th Century According to Contemporary Hebrew Sources* (New York, 1973); to situate and redefine some of the more debatable aspects, see Yerushlami, *From Spanish Court to Italian Ghetto*, pp. 30–42; and Josef Kaplan, 'The Portuguese Community of Amsterdam in the 17th Century. Between Tradition and Change' in A. Haim (ed.), *Society and Community* (Jerusalem, 1991), pp. 141–71.

32  García Ballester, 'Minorities and Medicine', p. 133.

33  For an account of the social infamy of having Jewish ancestry (supposed or real), and the far-reaching consequences in Hispanic society ot the time, see the pertinent reflections by Jaime Contreras, *Sotos contra Riquelmes. Regidores, inquisidores y criptojudíos* (Madrid, 1992), pp. 15–31.

34  The case of Bachelor Felipe de Nájera is, once again, highly enlightening with regard to these rivalries and conflicts: García Ballester, 'The Inquisition and minority medical practitioners', pp. 181–85.

35  A satisfactory general historical framework for the period in V. Palacio Atard et al., *La época de los primeros borbones I. La nueva monarquía y su posición en Europa (1700–1759)* (Madrid, 1987); and Giovanni Stiffoni et al., *La época de los primeros borbones II. La cultura española entre el Barroco y la Ilustración (1680–1759)* (Madrid, 1988).

36  Galende Díaz, *La crisis del siglo XVIII y la Inquisición española. El caso de la Inquisición toledana (1700–1820)* (Madrid, 1988), pp. 59–70.

37  An appropriate presentation of the historical conjuncture of the Inquisiton at the time is Teófanes Egido, 'La Inquisición en la España borbónica: el declive del Santo Oficio y la nueva coyuntura' in *Historia de la Inquisición en España y América*, vol. 1, pp. 1204–11; details of the scale of the last anti-Jewish persecution may be found in the same volume, pp. 1380–90.

38  These data are the fruit of our own calculations, based on collections of accounts of *autos-da-fé* kept in: BNM, Mss. 718, 8560, 9304, 10938 and 18659,21.

39  The best reconstruction of the trials and testimonies of inquisitorial repression of the Crypto-Jewish group in Madrid continues to be that offered by Caro Baroja, *Los judíos*, vol. 3, pp. 55–131.

40  José Mª. López Piñero, *Ciencia y técnica en la sociedad española de los siglos XVI y XVII* (Barcelona, 1979), pp. 387–433.

41  Alvar Martínez Vidal & José Pardo Tomás, '*In tenebris adhuc versantes*. La respuesta de los novatores españoles a la invectiva de Pierre Régis', *Dynamis*, 15 (1995), pp. 301–40 and the bibliography cited therein.

42  For the career of a royal physician: José Pardo Tomás & Alvar Martínez Vidal, 'El Tribunal del Protomedicato y los médicos reales (1665–1724): entre la gracia real y la carrera profesional', *Dynamis*, 16 (1996), pp. 59–89; for the particular case of Juan Muñoz y Peralta, ibid., pp. 88–89.

43  To evaluate comparatively the peculiarities and similarities between physicians and surgeons engaged in the Spanish Inquisition and those medical practitioners engaged in other European tribunals, more studies like those by Guido Ruggiero (quoted in note 4), and Esther Fischer-Homberger, *Medizin vor Gericht: Gerichtsmedizin von der Renaissance bis zur Aufklärung* (Bern, 1983) are needed.

# No Law, No Rights?
# Autopsy in Germany since 1800

*Cay-Rüdiger Prüll*

## Introduction

Today the links between law and medicine seem to be evident, at least in the Western World. Of course, every culture and society needs to regulate medicine. Contemporary discussions focus at securing the rights of the patient just as much as the rights of the physician. A growing tendency is the demand for comprehensive and unmisconstruable legal regulations framing diagnostic and therapeutic measures as well as the position of patients and practitioners.[1] In this respect, the pathological-anatomical examination of the corpse to detect the cause of death, that is performing an 'autopsy',[2] is a provocative topic in Germany. In 1993, reports about trading in body parts provoked a controversy about autopsy which, in spite of the declining number of autopsies, has still not come to an end.[3] There has been no special law in Germany to date which regulates the opening of a corpse for clinical examination, although there is a wide range of ideas as to whether or how to perform an autopsy.[4] The consent of relatives is required, in general, to perform an autopsy on a patient who has died in hospital. In 1987 about 60% of requests to perform an autopsy were refused by the relatives.

Autopsy legislation in Germany cannot be seen as being representative of the situation in other countries. There are different rules and regulations depending on the respective historical and cultural context. Although it is not possible to give a full account of the topic here, it can be illustrated by some examples. In Austria, based on the laws of Maria Theresia (1717–1780), her third successor, the Emperor Franz II (1768–1835) permitted autopsies to be conducted without the consent of the relatives in 1804. Therefore, Austria is one of the pioneer countries with respect to legislation in favour of autopsies where now the autopsy rate in major hospitals is close to 100%. Many countries tried to adopt the Austrian regulations, but later they were revised, leading to declining autopsy rates.[5] The regulations in the former German Democratic Republic (GDR) came very close to the Austrian case. An autopsy was 'demanded by law in cases of death before the age of 16 years, death in connection with pregnancy and birth, and death of individuals with transplanted organs or pacemakers. Also, when relatives express a desire for an autopsy, the law advises that such wishes be heeded.'[6] In general, consent of the relatives was not required to perform an autopsy. In France consent is not required, but relatives may object if they wish.[7] Besides the countries which prefer a compromise, Great Britain is at the opposite pole to Austria. In hospital deaths, the absolute permission of the relatives is required to perform an autopsy. The emphasis in the European States lies generally on legislation which requires the absolute consent of relatives. Remarkably, the question of legislation requiring relatives' consent or not, does not correlate with a decline or an increase in the rate of autopsy.[8]

The study will argue that no autopsy legislation is needed in Germany. Against the background of the history of autopsy in Germany since 1800, it will be shown that, in the case of autopsy, the human rights of patients as well as of practitioners and of pathologists can best be assured if there are no rigid legal regulations. The first section will deal with the rise and professionalisation of scientific pathology in the nineteenth and twentieth centuries and the resistance against autopsy. The second section will describe the legal position of autopsy in German history as well as efforts to solve the problem by legislation. The third will focus on the pathologist's consultation with the patient choosing the example of the German pathologist, Ludwig Aschoff (1866–1942), professor at the University of Freiburg in Germany from 1906 to 1936. The final section, in particular, will explain the fundamental problem and lead towards a conclusion.

## Pathological Anatomy, Scientific Medicine and the Resistance to Autopsy

IT IS WIDELY ACKNOWLEDGED that the significance of autopsies for medicine has been increasing ever since the mid-eighteenth century, when surgeons accepted the idea that it was necessary to have studied anatomy in order to perform operations more effectively. This also fostered pathological anatomy. In Paris around 1900, postmortem findings were routinely linked to those of living patients.[9] This development also influenced the introduction of autopsy in Germany. Although the process of institutionalisation of pathology at German universities was rather slow, the morgues of many hospitals after 1800 were used for autopsies to compare clinical and postmortem findings.[10] At the Charité-Hospital in Berlin, for example, physicians sometimes even competed with the first 'pathologists' for postmortem examinations. Nevertheless, there were no general routine activities in pathological anatomy in the first half of the nineteenth century: corpses of patients who had died in the wards were sent to the so-called *Prosektor* at irregular intervals. Mostly, there was no distinct separation between anatomy as such and pathological anatomy. At Berlin University, for example, the corpses of those who had died in hospital could be sent to the anatomy department for dissection or to the morgue for autopsy.[11] Furthermore, Romantic medicine in Germany, being prevalent at least between the end of the eighteenth century and about 1830, did not favour autopsies. Medicine was tied to philosophical concepts and was divided into several lines of thought. There was no unique concept of autopsy in serving medicine.[12] Against the backdrop of the work done in the field of the developmental history of man (*Naturgeschichte*), obtaining clinical knowledge when examining the patient seemed to be of paramount significance. Morbid anatomy seemed to be only of secondary importance.[13] Compared to pathological anatomy, the institutionalisation of normal anatomy developed significantly faster.[14] The increasing need for corpses in anatomy meant that dissection no longer was restricted to criminals and the unprivileged. As Ruth Richardson has shown for Britain, the victims of these new developments were the indigent poor. Not only in Britain, but also in Germany, the poor were mostly opposed to dissection.[15] The resistance also included resistance against autopsy. As this is a rather neglected topic in the historiography of pathology,[16] there is no detailed analysis of the resistance against autopsy in general or, specifically, in early nineteenth-century Germany. It can be assumed, according to the low degree of institutionalisation of morbid anatomy, that there was only sparse resistance in Germany during the first half of the last century.[17]

This situation changed as of 1850 when pathological anatomy became an integral part of the concept of scientific medicine. Above all, the Berlin pathologist, Rudolf Virchow (1821–1902), championed morbid anatomy as one of the most important cornerstones of scientific medicine. Virchow ascribed to autopsy a threefold function. First, to detect the cause of death, secondly, as a topic of medical education and, thirdly, as the basis of scientific research. Morbid anatomy was based on Virchow's principle of 'cellular pathology', viz. pathological morphological changes were attributed to processes in the cell. Thus, disease was seen as a process, being determined by the same rules as in physiological conditions. Disease was no distinguished *ens morbi*. Instead, it was the result of changed morphological structures of the human body, especially of the cell. The microscope, therefore, made it possible to extend organ and tissue pathology one step further.[18] Hence, autopsy became much more important for medical practice because morphological pathological changes could be detected more effectively by opening the corpse. On the other hand, pathology in Germany, because of its specialised function, underwent a process of separation from clinical practice. Until about 1900, every German university had its own chair and institute for pathology.[19]

In these changed conditions, clinical examination and research nurtured demands for more corpses. Therefore, resistance to autopsies became an increasing problem in Germany after 1850. This resistance was not organised but consisted mostly of individual actions. Although its history is difficult to pursue, there are enough indirect hints by clinicians and pathologists to suggest an interpretation. In 1861, Eduard Henoch (1820–1910), Professor of Medicine at the University of Berlin and from 1860 head of an outdoor clinic for children, reported on his work. He stated that 27 children had died between 12 January and 5 October 1860 and remarked that 'The people's prejudice against autopsy, which has been not erased until now, caused trouble also for ourselves. But we were successful in considering the diagnosis by autopsy even in half the cases.'[20] In 1886 Rudolf Virchow wrote that 'Every year the number of corpses, whose autopsy is rejected by the relatives, increases.'[21] Resistance against autopsy relied chiefly on religious and, moreover, on traditional beliefs in life after death.[22] The latter, in particular, covers a lot of beliefs and behavioural patterns dealing with death and dying and other problems related to this topic. Traditional beliefs do not make a clear distinction between life and death. A dead person is not believed to be dead, at least not immediately, but remains potentially and actively powerful. Therefore, it is absolutely necessary to obey certain rules and to perform certain rituals. These cover different stages on the way from the deathbed to the burial. First there was the wake, which was kept by several persons, who would tell each other horror stories or who would often laugh and make jokes.[23] The funeral procession was a kind of 'holy' act and there were fixed rules for the participants and their place in the order of the procession. The same applied to the pallbearer.[24] Since medieval times tolling bells when someone had died was a popular custom. The inhabitants of the village and maybe brothers of the deceased in monasteries would pray for the dead.[25] Especially in the case of the funeral repast, the deceased was assumed to be present and, therefore, it was obvious for everybody that the family had organised and paid for it. The family provided the last meal on behalf of the deceased. Also of importance were legal questions because the possessions of the dead person were taken on this earth.[26] There are many more examples such as the use of candles from the wake to the burial, which shows the mingling of religious and mystical popular beliefs.[27] They reveal a wide range of rituals which cannot be understood in rational terms. These rituals have mainly three aims. First, they claim to care for the deceased. The path from earth to the kingdom to come should be secured and should be relieved of burdens. Secondly, these rules claim to care for the survivors, who must protect themselves against the deceased who might return if anything has gone wrong with, for example, the possessions on earth or with the burial. Thirdly, death and dying are events with a potential for both good and evil magic as the corpse can be a source of magic power. Thus, rules and rituals preserving the integrity of the human corpse are absolutely necessary. Hence, in traditional terms, to perform an autopsy is to desecrate a corpse.[28] Several sources show that traditional beliefs had a strong impact on the German people in the nineteenth century. This impact waned at the end of the century, because working conditions had changed in the course of industrialisation and, in addition, the living conditions of the people had lost their medieval character since 1800. Around 1900, for example, increasing traffic and growing cities prevented major funeral processions from taking place. The influence of the government and of the Christian churches led to a restriction of popular rituals. They were now practised much more often by individuals than by a community of relatives and a lot of friends.[29] Yet, it would be a mistake to conclude that popular beliefs and traditional rituals have vanished totally. On the contrary, it can be stated that there is a certain set of behavioural patterns, which has been preserved from antiquity[30] to the twentieth century, at least in rural counties and districts.[31]

It seems that in nineteenth- and twentieth-century Germany resistance to autopsy was blocked or overthrown by the medical profession and its growing reputation as a scientific discipline in connection with the governments of the authoritarian states. In 1931, a woman complained about the autopsy that had been performed on her husband who had died in the Charité-Hospital in Berlin. In the mortuary she had lifted his shroud and had discovered the postmortem incisions. She wrote to the Ministry of Science and complained that the body had been cut up in crisscross fashion and that all of the organs had been removed. Furthermore, she claimed that her husband had been slaughtered alive for the sake of scientific interests. The woman informed the 'League of Human Rights'.[32] Her complaints seem to have been overly exaggerated and they were dismissed with the comment that the woman was mentally ill.[33] Nevertheless, her correspondence with the Ministry and the Charité physicians sheds some light on the attitudes of physicians and pathologists. The physicians claimed that there had been no objection to the autopsy when they had spoken to the relatives and that they had ordered the postmortem purely out of scientific interest.[34] Talking with the woman, the pathologist defended his work with the remark 'Do what you want to, if you take action against us. I have to protect my colleagues. Good afternoon!'[35] The woman noticed that the pathologist was very nervous, much more than she was herself.[36]

Another example from the Charité-Hospital in Berlin provides a far more detailed explanation of the difficulties encountered as a result of autopsies. In November 1929, a well-known French movie star and world champion wrestler of African origin died of leukaemia in the Charité-Hospital. Although his wife had definitely prohibited the autopsy, the corpse was dissected by the pathologist. Only by chance did she discover this blatant disregard of her husband's wishes for, dressed in black, she entered the dissection room of the Pathological Institute, ignoring any resistance in her way, and caught the pathologists at work.[37] The woman complained about the physicians and especially about the pathologist. Her husband, she said, had been a member of the Roman Catholic Church and, thus, had dreaded autopsy. The newspaper, *Berliner Zeitung*, reported on the case and published the widow's accusation. The headline about 'strange corpse rituals' in the Charité-Hospital reflected the previously mentioned traditional fears. The wife of the wrestler claimed damages for the unlawful mistreatment of her husband and the case was brought before the Prussian Ministry of Science. The Director of the Pathological Institute, Robert Rössle (1876–1956), defended himself. He said that he had told his assistant to perform an autopsy 'because clinically it was an especially important case and, because there was a written statement of clinical interest, the objection was invalid.' Rössle based his argument on section 9 of the Charité-Hospital's regulations pertaining to the handling of corpses, declaring that every corpse could be autopsied if it merited scientific interest. Consequently, the Ministry of Law dismissed the protest of the wrestler's wife.[38] This case shows the confrontation between scientific pathology's use of the human body for medical progress and lay attitudes on death and dying. Although this case was decided on the basis of certain regulations, the legal situation involving autopsy was less than clear.

## Autopsy and the Law

IN NINETEENTH- AND TWENTIETH-CENTURY Germany, the immediate decision as to how to deal with the corpse of a person who has died in hospital was based on the regulations of the individual hospital. These regulations included direct instructions for pathologists. However, they were not standardised and, thus, differed depending on locality and region, especially in respect to governmental decisions of the respective territorial states.[39] Moreover, such regulations did not remain constant but sometimes changed in these states according to social and political conditions. The Berlin Charité-Hospital may serve again as an example. In 1856, Rudolf Virchow succeeded in establishing a regulation that permitted autopsies if the relatives did not object within 18 hours.[40] In 1906, this regulation was further changed in favour of the pathologists. Autopsies were now permitted after 12 hours, if there was no objection.[41] A new regulation was introduced during the Revolution of 1918 which denoted a profound turn of direction. In December 1918, the democratic Ministry of Science ordered the Charité Administration to submit to every objection raised by the relatives against autopsy if the Charité Administration or the Director of the Pathological Institute could not succeed in persuading them to withdraw the protest.[42] Otto Lubarsch (1860–1933), at the time the pathologist holding the Virchow Chair, attacked the new regulation and argued that education and research in the field of pathology would be severely jeopardised. Lubarsch convinced his colleagues in the Medical Faculty to sign a petition against the order. The new regulation remained to be validated and there was no answer from the Ministry of Science. Lubarsch interpreted the Ministry's silence as approval of his measures. Without any consent, Lubarsch performed autopsies on many individuals who had been killed in the Berlin street fighting in the course of the revolution in January 1919. The Ministry now reminded Lubarsch to submit to the new regulation. Lubarsch objected to this once more by mentioning his duty in respect of medical education and research. He refused to accept the Ministry's admonition. Lubarsch received no answer from the Ministry and decided to proceed to perform autopsies without waiting for the consent of the relatives. In the following years Lubarsch was reminded of the need to acknowledge the Ministry's order several times and consequently he referred to his former response. In the last year of Lubarsch's directorship the regulation was finally changed.[43] Therefore, in 1929, Robert Rössle could insist on the restrictions for refusing dissection of a deceased relative and argued with section 9 of the Charité regulations. Evidently, these agreements between the pathologist and the hospital, which were influenced by the respective government of the individual territorial states, did not provide a definitive solution towards uniting the divergent positions.

In addition to the hospital regulations, there were also traditional regulations (*Leichenordnungen*) in individual German territorial states. In the course of the nineteenth century, these regulations were expanded to include specific instructions for the performance of inspections of the corpse (*Leichenschau*). After the foundation of the German Empire in 1871 the German parliament (*Reichstag*) debated the uniting of the different orders of the German territories and the enactment of general regulations without coming to any conclusions.[44] The regulations mainly provided general guidelines for delivering corpses to the funeral or for their use by anatomy departments or forensic medicine and were especially designed for medicolegal cases. Hence, they were not much more than bureaucratic orders. One such example is the Regulation promulgated by the State of Baden in 1904. It dealt with the corpses to be sent to the anatomical institutions of universities. The regulation defined those social groups, especially the poor, whose corpses could serve anatomical interests. Furthermore, this regulation stipulated the possibilities for the next of kin of preventing the dissection of a corpse, and for transporting corpses to anatomical institutions, and it also set out specific rules for the respective anatomical institutions and for funerals after dissection. It outlined the duties of the regional police and specified which documentation was necessary. Contemporary territorial regulations also mirror the public interest in plague prevention. Autopsy is not mentioned as the hospital's regulations were deemed to be the competent authority.[45]

To go to court regarding autopsy was only possible in terms of the general legal system of the individual German territorial states. In the German Empire, after 1871, the civil and the penal codes were used as a basis to implement a framework for regulating autopsies. A decisive factor in this respect was the German Imperial Court (*Deutsches Reichsgericht*) which set the trend in terms of case law. Between 1880 and 1945 it arbitrated on seven different cases dealing with the handling of corpses.[46] A case concerning the criminal court in September 1930 illustrates the dominant position of the German Imperial Court. The substitute Director of the University Clinic of Königsberg performed an autopsy upon a woman without obtaining the permission of her next of kin. The physician defended himself by emphasising that he was not aware of any objections to autopsy from the relatives. The Imperial Court discussed the case at remarkable length. The arguments focused on the question as to whether, in legal terms, a corpse is an object and consequently, whether the Director of the Clinic damaged the property of others. Based on court decisions in Germany since 1903, the Imperial Court rejected this attitude, partly because personal rights of the dead existed and still had to be acknowledged. Surprisingly, the Imperial Court did not want to decide whether a corpse is an object or not. Of decisive importance in this case was the fact that nobody was in possession of the corpse and, thus, it could not be defined as the property of another person. Hence, since the physician did not damage an object that was in the possession of another person, he was exonerated.[47]

This case is significant because the Imperial Court admitted that it could not clarify the legal situation. 'A specific legal regulation concerning the question discussed here is, of course, missing. But because of traditional manners and customs a legal position has habitually developed, treating the human corpse with exceptional legal premises because of its peculiarities. However that may be, no right of property concerning the corpse comes to exist by death alone.'[48] Nevertheless, there had developed a habitual right of the nearest relatives over the corpse of the beloved deceased. Thus, the relatives decide where the funeral will take place and how it will be performed and, above all, whether to reject any actions of unauthorised persons on the corpse. The Imperial Court confirmed in this way a legal construction, which was discussed previously by legal experts at that time. The corpse can be in custody of a person or an institution such as a hospital. The relatives have the authority, in the first instance, of acquisition of the corpse (*vorzugsweises Aneignungsrecht*). As the corpse is no one's property, those who are in custody of the corpse could not be charged for any useful measures in respect of the corpse, at least if they did not get the corpse under their control by an unauthorised infringement (*unbefugter Übergriff*). In addition, because the corpse is not an object, the pathologist cannot be accused of damaging an object while performing an autopsy. As the corpse is no longer living, a postmortem is not causing bodily harm (*Körperverletzung*). Thus, as the pathologist performs the postmortem for scientific reasons, opening a corpse is not being mischievous (*grober Unfug*). A physician who performs an autopsy, therefore, cannot be punished under the penal law.[49] Yet, even in 1928, the tendency was to acknowledge the consent of the deceased or of the relatives.[50]

Finally, it is not surprising that there was a certain number of pathologists who welcomed the period of the Third Reich when it was possible to perform autopsies with the help of the new government and without any control from the people. Corpses of victims of the 'Euthanasia' campaign and those of murdered political and racial persecutees in concentration camps were autopsied. One of the most well-known National Socialist pathologists is Berthold Ostertag (1895–1975). Between 1934 and 1945 he was head of the Pathological Institute of the Rudolf Virchow Hospital in Berlin. In the course of the 'Euthanasia' campaign he directed the autopsies of the murdered children from the paediatric psychiatric hospital 'Im Wiesengrund' in Berlin. Ostertag's career was successful because of his close contacts with important representatives of the National Socialist regime. He did not even hold back from slandering and criticising his colleagues. After 1945 he became Director of the Institute of Brain Research in Tübingen in Germany.[51] In contrast, the career of the SS physician and pathologist Robert Neumann (?1902) is almost unknown. He was one of the well-sponsored scholars of Robert Rössle. Neumann worked at the Pathological Institute of the Charité in Berlin between 1932 and 1935, and subsequently became head of the Pathological Institute of the Berlin-Moabit Hospital. There are severe hints that he conducted experiments on concentration camp inmates from Oranienburg near Berlin in this capacity and that he used the self-developed 'Histotom' to collect tissue specimens from the liver of living patients. Furthermore, Walter Poller, inmate and physician-secretary ('Arztschreiber') in the Buchenwald concentration camp, mentioned that (in 1939/40, the author) Neumann used his instrument even there. Neumann also would have conducted experiments with 'therapeutics' in Buchenwald and all of his victims would have died after the interventions. He would have performed autopsies after these victims had died. Neumann also worked in the Auschwitz concentration camp. From 1940 to at least 1943 he was head of the Pathological Institute of the German Medical Academy in Shanghai in China. In a court trial in 1948, Neumann was defended by a colleague who noted that 'it is not possible now to give an expert opinion about the real cause of death of the patients.' However, Neumann needed no help, because he could escape to Shanghai. In 1954, Neumann was a scientific assistant at the STADA pharmaceutical company in Tübingen in Germany.[52]

Besides this surely clandestine work of German pathologists, the official treatment of the German people with respect to autopsy worked in a similar manner to the outcome of the trials of the Imperial Court. But after 1933 there were also claims for legal solutions to perform autopsies without restrictions. In 1934 a Commission of the Medical Faculty of Berlin University tried to work out a new legal regulation to perform autopsies without any interference. Two of the six members of the commission were Robert Rössle and Fritz Lenz (1887–1976), the latter being head of the Department of Eugenics in the Kaiser-Wilhelm-Institute and Professor for Racial Hygiene at the University of Berlin from 1933. Whereas Lenz wanted to introduce regulations that enabled pathologists and physicians to enforce autopsies, Rössle was in fear of too much resistance from the relatives and, in an ambivalent mood, wanted to work with the existing regulations. Rössle wished to change conditions in favour of pathology more discreetly. He asked for the support of the Charité Administration and the physicians of the Charité-Hospital to use the possibilities of the hospital directives to increase the number of autopsies 'even against the will of the relatives'.[53] This did not seem to be successful as, in 1936, Rössle asked for an amendment to paragraph 9 of the Charité Regulations. Rössle intended to reduce any influence of the Charité Administration over the decision making with regard to the performing of autopsies. Surprisingly, this was prevented by the Ministry of Science, which feared that there would no longer be any possibility 'to consider individual cases'. Therefore, there were only minor undecisive changes to paragraph 9 in 1938.[54] In the period between 1933 and 1945 there were no changes in the law and no introduction of a new autopsy law.[55]

The legal situation concerning autopsies remained fully open to the ideas and wishes of both the pathologist and the relatives, depending on the case and the special setting in which the decision was made. This remains the case to the present day in the Federal Republic of Germany.[56] The legal situation was criticised in the past and is still being criticised, mainly by physicians and pathologists. Their claims are fostered by the interpretation of existing laws in the Federal Republic of Germany, because several trials took place because of 'illegal autopsies'.[57] Both physicians and pathologists want to have explicit instructions, rather than discussing their own scientific view and the arguments from traditional belief. These instructions, in their eyes, should give them autonomy over autopsies. The wish to receive some instructions is so urgently felt that, in 1979, the authors of one of the very few monographs on autopsy and its history even regretted that the Nazi period was not used to establish an autopsy law. 'Even legislation that was introduced in the Third Reich, and was sensible in respect of its subject matter and did not violate general human rights survived this period and either became a part of the legal measures constituting our democracy or did so after undergoing only unessential changes. Could it not have been done similarly as, for example, had been done with the Food, Animal Protection, Hunting and Animal Cadaver Elimination Acts, when enacting legislation on autopsies in the years of an elimination of parliament and oppositional social groups?'[58] Against the background of historical development the question should be asked. Is it wise to abandon discussion in favour of an unquestionable regulation? The example of Ludwig Aschoff shows that it is not.

## Talking to the Patient: Ludwig Aschoff (1866–1942)

THE PROFESSIONALISATION OF PATHOLOGY in the nineteenth century was influenced strongly by Rudolf Virchow's zealous fight for the success of scientific medicine in which he was supported also by other pioneers in this new way of handling pathology.[59] The post-Virchow generation was well acquainted with the aims of the founders of the discipline. Born in 1866, Ludwig Aschoff belonged to the following generation. He held the Chair of Pathology at the University of Freiburg from 1906 to 1936 and was to become the leading figure of German pathology in the first half of the twentieth century.[60] Like his colleagues, he was a strong advocate of autopsies. In World War I, he changed the discipline's scientific orientation towards military problems and created the 'war pathology' (*Kriegspathologie*). Aschoff planned to use the critical war situation to perform autopsies on every German soldier who had been killed in action. He not only intended to do routine work in morbid anatomy but also planned to examine the physical constitution of the German people (*Deutsches Volk*). Aschoff was successful in persuading nearly all of his colleagues holding important chairs of pathology in the German Empire to join his ambitious plan. During the war it had not been necessary to worry about obtaining permission from the relatives. Although resistance against autopsy is mentioned in publications on 'war pathology', it was easy to break this resistance because of the great distance between the theatres of war and the homelands.[61] During World War I Aschoff also secured a better position concerning autopsy regulations in Freiburg. In 1917, Aschoff was offered the chair at Rudolf Virchow's Institute in Berlin. He turned down this offer but gained some privileges in Freiburg. One of these was the decision of the municipal government to change the conditions for admission to the urban hospitals in favour of morbid anatomy. Autopsies could now be ordered by the hospital director in every case in which it seemed necessary to examine the disease and the cause of death. Aschoff now had, as he put it, 'favourable working conditions'.[62] They seemed to be so favourable that Georg Herzog (1884–1962), pathologist at the University of Giessen, sought Aschoff's advice and asked Aschoff to send him the regulations.[63]

Although Aschoff was a keen defender of autopsy in the Weimar Republic, he thought it important to keep in contact with the people. In October 1925 he gave a public lecture about the significance of autopsy and animal experimentation for the health of the people and for social welfare work. Aschoff admitted that autopsy belonged to those matters 'which are actually at odds with our natural human feeling',[64] thus consideration had to be taken of traditional belief. He accepted feelings of resistance which he had himself and which were also expressed by medical students. Traditional objections would be fundamental matters and Aschoff tried to find a form of harmonious coexistence between traditional beliefs and scientific medicine. Aschoff also promoted discussion. 'It is obvious that one can speak with total frankness only if the auditor has the necessary seriousness and the will to understand.'[65] Aschoff provided a broad description of autopsy, covering its significance for art and for the history of medicine. He carefully described the technique of opening the body and pointed out the differences between autopsy and dissection. 'The corpse is not cut up in crisscross fashion; instead, only one incision is necessary.'[66] After the orderly examination of the brain, the corpse would later show 'not the slightest trace of any change' in appearance.[67] Aschoff also emphasised the intactness of the body which should be preserved whenever possible. Thus, in spite of describing fully every aspect of the importance of autopsy, Aschoff explained the decision-making in favour of autopsy as a, sometimes, longer-lasting controversial process and, occasionally, as an agonising compromise. He illustrated this by describing various cases and admitted that sometimes it was hard work to convince the relatives to permit the autopsy. Aschoff's attitude was ambivalent, because he admitted objections to autopsy on anthropological grounds but also defended pathological anatomy. Aschoff's arguments aimed at an agreement between both sides, although he realised that there were limitations to his ideas. Anthropological factors were difficult to describe and to deal with, so that, even in 1934, Aschoff said that 'invisible powers' would often reject postmortems.[68]

## Conclusion

THE HISTORICAL DEVELOPMENT of autopsy in Germany is characterised by the rise of morbid anatomy from 1850 onwards. This is also accompanied by a resistance to autopsy, which became descriptive and manifest. This resistance made itself felt especially in the Weimar Republic but despite this development there was no legal regulation of autopsy in Germany. The legal situation remained open, fostering not only expert discussions but also a dispute between pathologists and the patient's relatives. The question of whether to perform an autopsy or not in our times appears to be an ethical problem. Pathologists and physicians claim that only by creating an autopsy law the dispute with relatives could be ended and the future of autopsy saved. Recently, a pathologist even asserted that ethical problems would result from a missing autopsy law.[69] This study would suggest that this is a misjudgement of the problems concerned with autopsy. In addition, it is not at all obvious whether an increasing number of autopsies leads to better medical care of the people.[70] On the contrary, pathologists would betray their own interests and influence as physicians by creating such a law, as there would no longer be the opportunity for individual decision-making appropriate to the respective cases.[71] Furthermore, historical formal regulations mainly restricted the possibilities for relatives to refuse an autopsy and any law would strengthen this situation. Undermining someone's right to refuse an autopsy cannot be justified by referring to the advantage of autopsy for society's health care,[72] because in doing so one would claim the right to commit an offence against individual rights, especially against the ethical principle of 'informed consent'.[73] It has to be concluded that legislation cannot solve the ethical problems with autopsy, above all when considering the historical dimensions of the problem. Therefore, there has been no autopsy law in Germany and problems have been solved on the basis of general aspects of the law.

The question remains about how to deal with decision-making in respect of performing autopsies. The dispute between pathologists and patients illustrates most clearly that it is not possible to cover the different viewpoints by legislation without violating the interests of both groups. The history of autopsy shows that this dispute is not a mere problem of being rational versus being irrational. Even morphological pathology cannot base its results on objectivity. Its representatives cannot furnish information about life after death. On the other hand, traditional beliefs do not consist only of insignificant measures. The fundamental problem comes from ethical grounds as both traditional beliefs and scientific medicine are two social constructs for explaining the world. Aschoff's concept of reconciliation does not work if discussions are restricted to persuading people that they must accept autopsies. Moreover, pathologists and patients or relatives of patients should start to discuss autopsy on equal terms.

No law, no rights? Human rights and the right to perform postmortems exist independently of any law and these rights are best preserved when every case is solved individually.[74] One remark in a comment on autopsy in the *Ärztliches Vereinsblatt* of 1928 describes the demands regarding postmortems even for our contemporary times. 'In practical life it will be constantly depend on reconciling scientific interests with the feelings of the relatives.'[75]

*I am grateful to the librarian of the Pathology Institute of the University of Freiburg, Mrs Elisabeth Demuth, for her generous help, and to Margareth Andergassen M.A. and Veronika Klaus for critical comments and assistance in translating the manuscript.*

# Notes

1  On the general history of legal medicine, see Michael Clark & Catherine Crawford (eds.), *Legal Medicine in History* (Cambridge, 1994).

2  For the reasons for performing postmortems, see Kenneth V. Iserson, *Death to Dust. What happens to dead Bodies?* (Tucson, 1994), pp. 109–67. Since August 1996, the American pathologist Edward O. Uthman has explained the procedure of autopsy for lay people on the internet. Edward O. Uthman, *The Routine Autopsy. The Procedure related in Narrative Form. A Guide for Screenwriters and Novelists* (uthman@neosoft.com).

3  Cf., 'Geplündert ins Grab', *Der Spiegel*, 49 (1993), 68–81; 'Lotsen der Therapie', *Der Spiegel*, 46 (1997), 208–12.

4  It was discussed without any effect to insert an autopsy law into the planned introduction of a law concerning organ transplantation: see, for example, Silvia Schattenfroh, 'Wiederverwertung nach dem Tode. Organentnahme und Transplantation', *Frankfurter Allgemeine Zeitung*, 1 March 1994, 14; Stefanie Heuer & Christoph Conrads, 'Aktueller Stand der Transplantationsgesetzgebung 1997', *Medizinrecht*, 15 (1997), 195–202; *Gesetz über die Spende, Entnahme und Übertragung von Organen* (Transplantationsgesetz-TPG); Hermann Christoph Kühn, 'Das neue deutsche Transplantationgesetz', *Medizinrecht*, 16 (1998), 455–61.

5  Einar Svendsen, 'Autopsy Legislation and Practice in Various Countries', *Archive of Pathology and Laboratory Medicine*, 111 (1987), 846–50, here p. 847. Svendsen describes the different conditions in various countries without giving any comparative statement about the effectiveness of autopsy regarding the respective countries. Concerning Austrian legislation, see also L. Sakr et al., 'Zur hohen Autopsierate in Wien', *Wiener klinische Wochenschrift*, 101 (1989), 511–14; G. Breitfellner, 'Die gesetzliche Sektionspflicht in österreichischen Krankenanstalten', *Der Pathologe*, 7 (1986), 62–63; W. Feigl & H. Leitner, 'Die hohe Autopsierate Österreichs und ihre Gründe', *Der Pathologe*, 7 (1986), 4–7.

6  Svendsen, 'Autopsy Legislation and Practice in Various Countries', 848.

7  Ibid.

8  Ibid., 849. For an international comparison of autopsy regulations see also Claudia Maria Brugger & Hermann Kühn, *Sektion der menschlichen Leiche. Zur Entwicklung des Obduktionswesens aus medizinischer und rechtlicher Sicht* (Stuttgart, 1979), pp. 100–13.

9  Concerning the 'Paris School of Medicine' see: Erwin H. Ackerknecht, *Medicine at the Paris Hospital, 1794–1848* (Baltimore, 1967); Toby Gelfand, *Professionalizing modern Medicine. Paris Surgeons and Medical Science and Institutions in the 18th Century* (Westport, CT, 1980); Gerald L. Geison (ed.), *Professions and the French State* (Philadelphia, 1984); William F. Bynum & Roy Porter (eds.), *William Hunter and the Eighteenth-Century Medical World* (Cambridge, 1985); Matthew Ramsey, *Professional and Popular Medicine in France, 1770–1830: The Social World of Medical*

*Practice* (Cambridge, 1988); Toby Gelfand, 'The History of the Medical Profession' in William F. Bynum & Roy Porter (eds.), *Companion Encyclopedia of the History of Medicine*, Vol. 2 (London & New York, 1993), 1119–50.

10 Cf. Hans-Heinz Eulner, *Die Entwicklung der medizinischen Spezialfächer an den Universitäten des deutschen Sprachgebietes* (Stuttgart, 1970), pp. 95–110.

11 See Peter Krietsch, 'Zur Geschichte der Prosektur der Charité Berlin, 1. Gründung der Prosektur und Philipp Phoebus als erster Prosektor', *Zentralblatt für allgemeine Pathologie und pathologische Anatomie*, 136 (1990), 377–87; ibid., 'Zur Geschichte der Prosektur der Charité Berlin, 2. Mitteilung. Robert Friedrich Froriep, Prosektor der Charité von 1833 bis 1864', *Zentralblatt für allgemeine Pathologie und pathologische Anatomie*, 136 (1990), 729–38.

12 For German romantic medicine, see Hans-Uwe Lammel, *Nosologische und therapeutische Konzeptionen in der romantischen Medizin* (Abhandlungen zur Geschichte der Medizin und der Naturwissenschaften, Vol. 59) (Husum, 1990); Dietrich v. Engelhardt, 'Romantische Mediziner', in Dietrich v. Engelhardt & Fritz Hartmann (eds.), *Klassiker der Medizin, vol. 2, Von Philippe Pinel bis Viktor von Weizsäcker* (Munich, 1991), 95–118.

13 See, for example, Johanna Bleker, 'Johann Lukas Schönlein (1793–1864)' in ibid., 81–94. Here are no remarks on autopsy; only very few comments in: idem, *Die Naturhistorische Schule 1825–1845. Ein Beitrag zur Geschichte der Klinischen Medizin in Deutschland* (Stuttgart, New York, 1981); idem, Eva Brinkschutte & Pascal Grosse (eds.), *Kranke und Krankheiten in Juliusspital zu Würzburg 1819–1829. Zur frühen Geschichte des Allgemeinen Krankenhauses in Deutschland* (Abhandlungen zur Geschichte der Medizin und der Naturwissenschaften, vol. 72) (Husum, 1995).

14 Eulner, *Die Entwicklung der medizinischen Spezialfächer*, pp. 495, 506.

15 Ruth Richardson, *Death, Dissection and the Destitute* (London, 1988); Christel Heckhausen, *Anatomen und Anatomie im Urteil der Öffentlichkeit seit 1500* (Berlin, Diss.Med.Fak., 1966), pp. 65–75; Klaus D. Mörike, *Geschichte der Tübinger Anatomie* (Tübingen, 1988); Andreas-Holger Maehle, 'Einstellungen zur Sektion der menschlichen Leiche im 17. und 18. Jahrhundert', *Niedersächsisches Ärzteblatt*, 17 (1991), 1–5.

16 Cf. further literature such as David Harley, 'Political Post-mortems and Morbid Anatomy in Seventeenth-century England', *Social History of Medicine*, 7 (1994), 1–28. In general works about the history of pathology, resistance against autopsy is not mentioned or dealt with only randomly. Russel C. Maulitz, 'The Pathological Tradition' in Bynum & Porter (eds.), *Companion Encyclopedia of the History of Medicine*, Vol. 1, (London & New York, 1993), 169–91; George J. Cunningham, *The History of British Pathology* (Bristol, 1993); Axel Bauer, *Die Krankheitslehre auf dem Weg zur naturwissenschaftlichen Morphologie. Pathologie auf den Versammlungen Deutscher Naturforscher und Ärzte von 1822–1872* (Stuttgart, 1989); Russel C. Maulitz, *Morbid appearances. The anatomy of pathology in the early nineteenth century* (Cambridge, 1987); Teizo Ogawa (ed.), *History of Pathology*. Proceedings of the 8th

international Symposium on the comparative history of Medicine – East and West (18–24 September 1983, Susono-shi, Shizuoka, Japan) (Tokyo, 1983); William Derek Foster, _Pathology as a profession in Great Britain and the early history of the Royal College of Pathologists_ (London, 1983); idem, A _short History of Clinical Pathology_ (Edinburgh/London, 1961); Edwin B. Krumbhaar, _Pathology_ (Clio Medica XIX) (New York, 1937, repr. 1962); Esmond R. Long, A _History of American Pathology_ (Springfield, 1962); idem, A _History of Pathology_ (Baltimore, 1928, New York, 1965); Walther Fischer & Georg B. Gruber, _Fünfzig Jahre Pathologie in Deutschland_ (Stuttgart, 1949); Edgar Goldschmid, _Entwicklung und Bibliographie der pathologisch-anatomischen Abbildung_ (Leipzig, 1925).

17 See Claudia Maria Brugger, _Zur Entwicklung des Obduktionswesens aus medizinischer und rechtlicher Sicht_ (Thesis Med. Fac. Heidelberg, 1977); Brugger & Kühn, _Sektion der menschlichen Leiche_, p. 86.

18 For Virchow, see Erwin H. Ackerknecht, _Rudolf Virchow. Arzt, Politiker, Anthropologe_ (Stuttgart, 1957), Manfred Vasold, _Rudolf Virchow. Der große Arzt und Politiker_ (Stuttgart, 1988). See, furthermore, Ludwig Buhl, _Ueber die Stellung und Bedeutung der pathologischen Anatomie_ (Munich, 1863).

19 For the institutionalisation of German pathology, see Irmgard Hort, _Die Pathologischen Institute der deutschsprachigen Universitäten (1850–1914)_ (Thesis Med. Fac. Cologne, 1987); Johannes Pantel & Axel Bauer, 'Die Institutionalisierung der Pathologischen Anatomie im 19. Jahrhundert an den Universitäten Deutschlands, der deutschen Schweiz und Österreichs', _Gesnerus_, 47 (1990), 303–28.

20 'Das noch immer nicht getilgte Vorurtheil des Publicums gegen Sectionen trat auch uns störend entgegen; doch gelang es uns wenigstens in der Hälfte dieser Fälle, die Diagnose durch die Autopsie zu bestätigen'; see Eduard Henoch, _Beiträge zur Kinderheilkunde_ (Berlin, 1861), pp. 1–2, see the quotation on p. 2.

21 'Mit jedem Jahre nimmt die Zahl der Leichen zu, welche durch die Angehörigen der Sektion entzogen werden'. See Rudolf Virchow, 'Das Pathologische Institut' in Albert Guttstadt (ed.), _Die naturwissenschaftlichen und medicinischen Staatsanstalten Berlins. Festschrift für die 59. Versammlung deutscher Naturforscher und Aerzte_ (Berlin, 1886), pp. 288–300, esp. p. 295.

22 Also today there are approaches, even from the clerical side, to reduce the problem of resistance to autopsies on mere religious feelings. This argument is far too short. See Franz Böckle, 'Pietät oder Nächstenliebe? Zur sittlichen Bewertung der medizinischen Obduktion', _Der Pathologe_, 4 (1983), 1–2.

23 Peter Löffler, _Studien zum Totenbrauchtum in den Gilden, Bruderschaften und Nachbarschaften Westfalens vom Ende des 15. bis zum Ende des 19. Jahrhunderts_ (Forschungen zur Volkskunde, Vol. 47) (Münster, 1975), pp. 58–74; Friederike Schepper-Lambers, _Beerdigungen und Friedhöfe im 19. Jahrhundert in Münster_ (Beiträge zur Volkskultur in Nordwestdeutschland, Vol. 73), pp. 18–19.

24 Ibid., pp. 24–28; Löffler, _Studien zum Totenbrauchtum in den Gilden_, pp. 75–151, esp. p. 75.

25 Ibid., pp. 152–86, esp. p. 153; Schepper-Lambers, *Beerdigungen und Friedhöfe im 19. Jahrhundert in Münster*, pp. 77–79.

26 Löffler, *Studien zum Totenbrauchtum in den Gilden*, pp. 247–291, esp. pp. 247–48.

27 Ibid., pp. 187–223.

28 Cf. Cay-Rüdiger Prüll, 'Der Umgang mit der menschlichen Leiche: Medizinhistorischer Überblick' (Lecture presented at the conference 'Zum Umgang mit der Leiche in der Medizin' of the AEM (*Akademie für Ethik in der Medizin e.V.*) on 8–9 July 1994 in Heidelberg); idem, 'Die Sektion als letzter Dienst am Vaterland. Die deutsche "Kriegspathologie" im Ersten Weltkrieg' in Wolfgang U. Eckart & Christoph Gradmann (eds.), *Die Medizin und der Erste Weltkrieg* (Neuere Medizin- und Wissenschaftsgeschichte. Quellen und Studien, Vol. 3) (Pfaffenweiler, 1996), 155–82, esp. 175–76. In respect of cultural-historical and anthropological resistance against autopsy see the articles in the '*Handwörterbuch des Deutschen Aberglaubens*', edited with the collaboration of E. Hoffmann-Krayer and many colleagues by Hanns Bächtold-Stäubli (*Handwörterbuch zur deutschen Volkskunde, Abt.1: Aberglaube*), Vols 1–10 (Berlin 1927–1942); above all the articles 'Tote (der)' by Paul Geiger, in ibid., Vol. VIII (Berlin & Leizig, 1936–1937), col. 1019–1034; 'Leiche' by Paul Geiger in ibid., Vol. V (Berlin & Leipzig, 1932–1933), col. 1024–1060; 'Leichenschändung' by Paul Geiger in ibid., Vol. V (Berlin & Leipzig, 1932–1933), col. 1093–1094.

29 Löffler, *Studien zum Totenbrauchtum in den Gilden*, pp. 292–97; Schepper-Lambers, *Beerdigungen und Friedhöfe im 19. Jahrhundert in Münster*, pp. 133–37.

30 In respect of burial practices, death rituals and resistance against autopsy in the ancient world, see Fridolf Kudlien, 'Antike Anatomie und menschlicher Leichnam', *Hermes*, 97 (1969), 78–94; Heinrich von Staden, 'The Discovery of the Body: Human Dissection and its cultural Contexts in Ancient Greece', *The Yale Journal of Biology and Medicine*, 65 (1992), 223–41; concerning the preservation of ancient rituals in modern Greece see Margaret Alexiou, *The Ritual Lament in Greek Tradition* (Cambridge, 1974).

31 In historical perspective see Hanns Bächtold, *Deutscher Soldatenbrauch und Soldatenglaube* (Strasbourg, 1917); E.M. Kronfeld, *Der Krieg im Aberglauben und Volksglauben. Kulturhistorische Beiträge* (Munich, 1917); Gotthold Bohne, 'Das Recht zur klinischen Leichensektion', in *Festgabe für Richard Schmidt. Zu seinem siebzigsten Geburtstag am 19. Januar 1932 überreicht von Verehrern und Schülern* (Leipzig, 1932), 105–76; Günther Oberhoff, *Über die Rechtswidrigkeit und Strafbarkeit klinischer Leichensektionen* (Thesis Fac.Law Erlangen) (Emsdetten, 1935), p. 5; Tamás Grynaeus, 'Weiterleben der heilenden Volksbräuche und -glauben in einem neugesiedelten Dorf in Ungarn', *Curare*, 3 & 4 (1993), 191–92; Christian Probst, 'Die Religiosität des Landvolks im Urteil der Ärzte. Aus den Landes- und Volksbeschreibungen der bayerischen Amtsärzte um 1860', *Die Medizinische Welt*, 45 (1994), 152–56. See in the case of contemporary ideas in respect of autopsy, for example 'Comments within the trade-of-organ discussion in Germany in 1993', *Der Spiegel*, 51 (1993), 10 & 12. The corpse is dealt with as a living person in Georg

Heym, 'Die Sektion' in Heinz Rölleke (ed.), *Georg Heym Lesebuch: Gedichte, Prosa, Träume, Tagebücher* (Munich, 1984), 181–83. Countless movies and pieces of literature, even today, deal with the ressurection of dead persons because of their mistreatment in life.

32  'Liga für Menschenrechte', see Complaint Th.K. to the Ministry of Science, Berlin, 20 July 1932 (3 pages) in *Verfahren bei der Behandlung der in dem Charité-Krankenhause Verstorbenen, insbesondere Sektionen; Dezember 1929 bis März 1938*, Bundesarchiv Berlin. Abteilung Lichterfelde (BArchiv Berlin), Reichsministerium für Wissenschaft, Erziehung und Volksbildung (REM), Vol. 2, No. 2697, no page numbers; A.K. to the Minister of Science, Berlin, no date (pp. 1–3), in ibid.

33  See the respective letters in ibid.

34  Prof. Kauffmann, Dr Stroebe, II. Medical Clinic of the Charité-Hospital to the Charité-Administration, Berlin, 7 December 1931, (2 pages); The Ministry of Science to Mrs K., Berlin, 26 January 1932 (2 pages), in ibid.

35  'Unternehmen Sie gegen uns was Sie wollen, ich muß meine Kollegen schützen. Guten Tag', see Mrs A.K. to the Ministry of Science, no date, pp. 3–4 in ibid.

36  Ibid., pp. 3–4.

37  The Ministry of Science, Notice, Berlin, 27 November 1929, in ibid.

38  'da es sich um einen klinisch besonders wichtigen Fall handelt und der Einspruch bei dem schriftlich geäußerten klinischen Interesse dadurch hinfällig geworden war', see Robert Rössle to the Charité-Administration, Berlin, 27 November 1929, in ibid. See furthermore The Ministry of Science, Notice, Berlin, 27 November 1929; Max Lenz, 'Sonderbarer Leichenkult in der Charité. Obduktion trotz Einspruchs der Hinterbliebenen. "Klinisches Interesse geht vor."', *Neue Berliner Zeitung*, No. 274, Vol. 11, Friday, 22 November 1929; Charité-Administration, Ordnung über das Verfahren bei der Behandlung der in dem Charitékrankenhause Verstorbenen, Berlin, 10 January 1928, in ibid.

39  Oberhoff, *Über die Rechtswidrigkeit und Strafbarkeit klinischer Leichensektionen*, p. 37.

40  Wilhelm Doerr, 'Geleitwort' in Brugger & Kühn, *Sektion der menschlichen Leiche*, VII/VIII, here VIII.

41  Johannes Orth, Das Pathologische Institut zu Berlin, *Berliner Klinische Wochenschrift*, 43 (1906), 817–26, esp. 824.

42  Otto Lubarsch, *Ein bewegtes Gelehrtenleben. Erinnerungen und Erlebnisse. Kämpfe und Gedanken* (Berlin, 1931), p. 340.

43  Ibid., pp. 340–41.

44  Roland Walter, *Die Leichenschau und das Sektionswesen. Grundzüge der Entwicklung von ihren Anfängen bis zu den Bemühungen um eine einheitliche Gesetzgebung* (Thesis Med.Fac. Düsseldorf, 1971), pp. 62–91.

45  Vorschriften über die Ablieferung von Leichen an die anatomischen Anstalten, Karlsruhe 1904, pp. 1–11, in *Die Vornahme von Sektionen betreffend 1905/1906*, Med.Fak. B 37, No. 416, Universitätsarchiv Freiburg i.Br.

46 'Genügt es, wenn die ärztlichen Sachverständigen, welche sich bei Abgabe ihres
Gutachtens zugleich über ihre Wahrnehmungen betreffs des thatsächlichen
Leichenbefundes, der vorgefundenen Verletzungen u.s.w. ausgelassen haben, nur als
Sachverständige, nicht auch als Zeugen beeidigt werden?' in *Entscheidungen des
Reichsgerichts in Strafsachen*, Vol. 2 (Leipzig, 1880), 389–90; '5. Enthält die in der
Hauptverhandlung mündlich erfolgte Bestätigung eines auf den Sektionsbefund
gegründeten schriftlichen Gutachtens seitens der begutachtenden Ärzte zugleich
die mündlich erfolgte Bestätigung des verlesenen Protokolls über die Leichenöffnung?', '6. Darf das Protokoll über die Leichenöffnung, im Gegensatz zu
demjenigen über die Leichenschau, in der Hauptverhandlung verlesen werden?',
'7. Ist der Grund der Verlesung im Sitzungsprotokolle anzugeben?' in ibid., Vol. 2
(Leipzig, 1880), 153–60; '1. Was ist unter "Beiseiteschaffen" eines Leichnams zu
verstehen?', '2. Wann ist ein Leichnam "ohne Vorwissen der Behörde" beiseite
geschafft?' in ibid., Vol. 28 (Leipzig, 1896), 119–22; 'Kann in dem unbefugten
Herausnehmen einer Leiche aus der noch offenen Gruft, in der sie beigesetzt war,
ein Vergehen gegen § 168 St.G.B.'s gefunden werden?' in ibid., Vol. 28 (Leipzig,
1896), 139–41; 'Der Veranstalter einer "politischen Demonstration" bei einem
Leichenbegängnis als Veranstalter eines nicht gewöhnlichen Leichenbegängnisses'
in ibid., Vol. 45 (Berlin & Leipzig, 1912), 85–88; 'Vorraussetzungen für die
Lesbarkeit eines Leichenschauprotokolls' in ibid., Vol. 53 (Berlin & Leipzig, 1920),
348–49; 'Kann an einem menschlichen Leichnam durch unbefugte Leichenöffnung
Sachbeschädigung begangen werden?' in *Entscheidungen des Reichsgerichts in
Strafsachen*, Vol. 64 (Berlin & Leipzig, 1931), 313–16.

47 Ibid., 313–16.

48 'An einer ausdrücklichen gesetzlichen Regelung der zur Entscheidung stehenden
Frage fehlt es freilich. Es hat sich aber gewohnheitsrechtlich auf Grund der
Volkssitten und =Gebräuche eine Rechtslage herausgebildet, nach welcher der
Leichnam des Menschen um seiner Besonderheiten willen eine eigenartige
rechtliche Behandlung erfährt, jedenfalls aber an ihm nicht schon durch den Tod
ein Eigentumsrecht zur Entstehung gelangt', see ibid., 315.

49 Hans Georg Bauer, *Die Behandlung des menschlichen Leichnams im geltenden deutschen
Recht* (Dresden, 1929), pp. 20–27. The decisive paragraphs in the German penal
law (*Strafgesetzbuch*) concerning autopsies are § 168 (theft of a corpse), § 367
(removing parts of the corpse). Furthermore, the following paragraphs play a certain
role: § 303 (damaging an object), § 223 ff (bodily harm), § 360.11 (being up to
mischief). See Oberhoff, *Über die Rechtswidrigkeit und Strafbarkeit klinischer
Leichensektionen*, pp. 6–29; Heinrich Seesemann, 'Ist eine heimliche Leichensektion
strafbar?', *Ärztliches Vereinsblatt*, 60 (1931), 45–46; Bohne, *Das Recht zur klinischen
Leichensektion.*

50 Heinrich Seesemann, 'Ist eine heimliche Leichensektion strafbar?', *Ärztliches
Vereinsblatt*, 55 (1928), 721.

51 Jürgen Peiffer, *Hirnforschung im Zwielicht: Beispiele verführbarer Wissenschaft aus
der Zeit des Nationalsozialismus. Julius Hallervorden – H.J. Scherer–Berthold Ostertag*

(Abhandlungen zur Geschichte der Medizin und der Naturwissenschaften, Vol. 79) (Husum, 1997), pp. 72–96; Christian Pross, 'Die "Machtergreifung" im Kranken-haus', in Johanna Bleker & Norbert Jachertz (eds.), *Medizin im "Dritten Reich"* (Cologne, 1993²), pp. 97–108, esp. p. 105; Götz Aly, 'Der saubere und der schmutzige Fortschritt', in idem (ed.), *Reform und Gewissen. "Euthanasie" im Dienst des Fortschritts* (Beiträge zur nationalsozialistischen Gesundheits- und Sozialpolitik 2) (Berlin, 1985), pp. 9–78, esp. pp. 64–71; Martina Krüger, 'Kinderfachabteilung Wiesengrund. Die Tötung behinderter Kinder in Wittenau', in *Totgeschwiegen 1933–1945. Zur Geschichte der Wittenauer Heilstätten. Seit 1957 Karl-Bonhoeffer-Nervenklinik*, edited by the Arbeitsgruppe zur Erforschung der Geschichte der Karl-Bonhoeffer-Nervenklinik, scientific adviser, Götz Aly (Berlin, 1989²), pp. 151–76; Cay-Rüdiger Prüll, *Medizin am Toten oder am Lebenden? – Pathologie in Berlin und in London 1900 bis 1945* (typewritten manuscript), forthcoming.

52  Hessisches Staatsministerium. Der Minister für politische Befreiung. Spruch-kammer Darmstadt-Lager, an Emil Carlebach, Vereinigung der Verfolgten des Nazi-Regimes (VVN), Darmstadt, 31 May 1948; ""Arztschreiber Poller gegen SS-Arzt Neumann", *Der Tagesspiegel*, 23 September 1948, newspaper cutting (see the quotation here, 'man könnte heute kein Gutachten mehr über die wahre Todesursache der Patienten abgeben'); Oskar Holewa an das Hessische Staatsministerium; der Minister für politische Befreiung. Spruchkammer Darmstadt-Lager, 26 April 1948; Das Hessische Staatsministerium; der Minister für politische Befreiung. Spruchkammer Darmstadt-Lager, an Staatskommissar Auerbach beim Sonderministerium für politische Befreiung, München, Darmstadt, 4 March 1948 in Bundesarchiv Koblenz, Aussenstelle Dahlwitz-Hoppegarten, *Akten des Ministeriums für Staatssicherheit der ehem. DDR, ZM 854 A. 16* (concerning Robert Neumann); Besetzung der Konzentrationslager in Bundesarchiv Berlin, Ordner SS, SL 19a, S.32; Walter Poller, *Arztschreiber in Buchenwald. Bericht des Häftlings 996 aus Block 39* (Hamburg, 1947), pp. 219–23; Ernst Klee, *Auschwitz, die NS-Medizin und ihre Opfer* (Frankfurt/M., 1997), pp. 36, 48 & 55; Christian Pross, 'Die "Machtergreifung" am Krankenhaus' in Christian Pross & Rolf Winau (eds.), *Nicht mißhandeln!* (Stätten der Geschichte Berlins, Vol. 5) (Berlin, 1984), pp. 180–205, esp. pp. 195–96. See further information on sources concerning Neumann in Prüll, *Medizin am Toten oder am Lebenden?*

53  Der Dekan der Medizinischen Fakultät der Universität Berlin an die Mitglieder der Kommission zur Beratung über die Schwierigkeiten, die für die Vornahme von Sektionen vorliegen (pencil notes of the Dean of the Medical Faculty of the University of Berlin), Berlin, 4 July 1934; Fritz Lenz to the Dean of the Medical Faculty, Berlin, 18 July 1934; Robert Rössle to the Dean of the Medical Faculty of the University of Berlin, Berlin, 18 July 1934 (see the quotation 'selbst gegen den Willen der Angehörigen') in *Akte betr. Sektionen. Leichenmangel (1934–1946)*, Universitätsarchiv der Humboldt-Universität Berlin, Medizinische Fakultät – Dekanat –, No. 281, p. 1–4.

54 The Director of Administration of the Charité-Hospital to the Ministry of Science, Berlin, 28 May 1936; Ministry of Science, Notice of Ministerialrat Breuer, no date (see the quotation here fears that 'kaum noch eine strenge Prüfung des Einzelfalles stattfindet'); The Director of Administration of the Charité-Hospital to the Ministry of Science, Berlin, 15 February 1938 in *Verfahren bei der Behandlung der in dem Charité-Krankenhause Verstorbenen, insbesondere Sektionen, Dezember 1929 bis März 1938*, in Bundesarchiv Berlin, Reichsministerium für Wissenschaft, Erziehung und Volksbildung, Bd.2, No. 2697. See further information in Prüll, *Medizin am Toten oder am Lebenden?*

55 Brugger & Kühn, *Sektion der menschlichen Leiche*, p. 124.

56 For contemporary law in the Federal Republic of Germany regarding autopsy see W. Eisenmenger, P. Betz & R. Penning, 'Arztrechtliche Fragen in der Pathologie I. Zur Rechtslage bei klinischen Sektionen', *Der Pathologe*, 12 (1991), 126–30.

57 'Prozesse wegen "rechtswidriger klinischer Sektionen"' see Brugger & Kühn, *Sektion der menschlichen Leiche*, p. 120.

58 'Selbst im 3. Reich eingeführte, von der Sache her sinnvolle Gesetze, die nicht gegen allgemeine Menschenrechte verstießen, überdauerten diese Zeit und wurden zu einem Bestandteil des Rechtsgutes unserer Demokratie oder erfuhren nur unwesentliche Änderungen. Hätte es bei der Schaffung eines in diesen Jahren bei Ausschaltung des Parlamentes und widersprüchlicher Interessengruppen leicht einzuführenden Sektionsrechtes nicht ähnlich gehen können wie beispielsweise mit dem Lebensmittel-, dem Tierschutz-, einem Jagdgesetz und einem Gesetz über die Beseitigung von gefallenen (verendeten) Tierkörpern?', see ibid., p. 124.

59 Ackerknecht, *Virchow*, pp. 1–33; Volker Becker, *Pathologie. Beständigkeit und Wandel* (Berlin, Heidelberg etc., 1996), pp. 7–18.

60 For Aschoff's life, see Ludwig Aschoff, *Ein Gelehrtenleben in Briefen an die Familie* (Freiburg i.Br., 1966); Franz Büchner, 'Ludwig Aschoff' in Johannes Vincke (ed.), *Freiburger Professoren des 19. und 20. Jahrhunderts* (Freiburg i.Br., 1957), 11–20; idem, 'Gedenkrede auf Ludwig Aschoff, gehalten bei der Gedenkfeier der Universität Freiburg am 5 Dezember 1943' (*Feldpostbrief der Medizinischen Fakultät der Universität Freiburg/Brsg.*, No. 4) (Freiburg, 1943), 1–24; Eduard Seidler, 'Pathologie in Freiburg', *Beiträge zur Allgemeinen Pathologie und pathologischen Anatomie*, 158 (1976), 9–22; idem, *Die Medizinische Fakultät der Albert-Ludwigs-Universität Freiburg im Breisgau. Grundlagen und Entwicklungen* (Berlin, Heidelberg etc., 1991), pp. 207–10, 270–72 & 333–34; Dorothea Buscher, *Die wissenschafts-theoretischen, medizinhistorischen und zeitkritischen Arbeiten von Ludwig Aschoff* (Thesis Med.Fac. Freiburg i.Br., 1980); Walther Fischer, 'Ludwig Aschoff. 1866–1942', in Hugo Freund & Alexander Berg (eds.), *Geschichte der Mikroskopie. Leben und Werk grosser Forscher*, Vol. 2, *Medizin* (Frankfurt/M., 1964), 13–21; Rudolf Meessen, *Die Freiburger Pathologie, ihre Entstehung und Fortentwicklung* (Thesis Med.Fac. Freiburg i.Br., 1975), pp. 19–31; Cay-Rüdiger Prüll, 'Aschoff, Ludwig' in Wolfgang U. Eckart & Christoph Gradmann (eds.), *Ärzte-Lexikon. Von der Antike bis zum 20. Jahrhundert* (Munich, 1995), 24–25; Lazare Benaroyo, 'Pathology and

the Crisis of German Medicine (1920–1930): A Study of Ludwig Aschoff's Case',
in Cay-Rüdiger Prüll in collaboration with John Woodward (ed.), *Pathology in the
19th and 20th Centuries. The Relationship between Theory and Practice* (Sheffield,
1997), 101–13; Susan Gross Solomon & Jochen Richter (eds.), *Ludwig Aschoff.
Vergleichende Völkerpathologie oder Rassenpathologie. Tagebuch einer Reise durch
Rußland und Transkaukasien (Neuere Medizin und Wissenschaftsgeschichte. Quellen
und Studien*, vol. 7) (Pfaffenweiler, 1998); Cay-Rüdiger Prüll, 'Pathologie und
Politik – Ludwig Aschoff (1866–1942) und Deutschlands weg ins Dritte Reich',
*History and Philosophy of the Life Sciences*, 19 (1997), 331–68.

61  Cf. Prüll, 'Die Sektion als letzter Dienst am Vaterland', 155–82.

62  'günstige(n) Arbeitsbedingungen', see Ludwig Aschoff to Karl Flügge, Dean of the
Medical Faculty, Berlin, Freiburg, 27 July 1917 in *Estate Ludwig Aschoff, div. V/2.
Vor und im Ersten Weltkrieg*, no page numbers, Institut für Geschichte der Medizin,
Freiburg i.Br. I would like to thank Professor Jürgen Aschoff for generously placing
major parts of his father's estate (Ludwig Aschoff (1866–1942)) and offprint
collection at the disposal of the Institute of the History of Medicine at the
University of Freiburg for scientific research. Both sets of writing have been
entrusted to the care of the Institute for the History of Medicine in Freiburg. See
furthermore Meessen, *Die Freiburger Pathologie*, p. 23.

63  Georg Herzog to Ludwig Aschoff, Giessen, 19.12.1928 in *Estate Ludwig Aschoff, div.
VI/2. Wissenschaftliche Korrespondenz. Deutschland 1.3.1927–31.12.1929*, no page
numbers.

64  'Dinge, "die unserem natürlichen menschlichen Empfinden eigentlich entgegen-
stehen, mit denen wir uns nicht ohne weiteres abfinden können"', see Ludwig
Aschoff, 'Über die Bedeutung der Leichenöffnungen und des Tierexperiments für
die Volksgesundheit und die soziale Wohlfahrtspflege', in *Wissenschaft und
Werktätiges Volk* (Verlag der Notgemeinschaft der Deutschen Wissenschaft),
151–85, here 151.

65  'Es ist ganz selbstverständlich, daß man mit voller Offenheit nur dann sprechen
kann, wenn man bei der Zuhörerschaft den nötigen Ernst und auch den Willen zum
Verstehen findet', see ibid., 153.

66  'Die Leiche wird keineswegs kreuz und quer zerschnitten, sondern es ist nur ein
einziger Schnitt, der notwendig ist', see ibid., 158.

67  'nicht die geringste Spur einer Veränderung', see ibid., 159.

68  'unsichtbare Kräfte', see Ludwig Aschoff to Ernst Rüdin, Freiburg, 26 September
1934 in *Estate Ludwig Aschoff, VI/8, Wissenschaftliche Korrespondenz Deutschland
1.1.1934–31.10.1934, II: L–Z*, no page numbers.

69  Udo Löhrs, 'Ethik in der Pathologie – Anmerkungen', in Dietrich v. Engelhardt
(ed.), *Ethik im Alltag der Medizin. Spektrum der Disziplinen zwischen Forschung und
Therapie* (Basel, Boston & Berlin, 1997), 61–74, esp. 67.

70  See, for example, Svendsen, 'Autopsy Legislation and Practice in Various
Countries', 846–50.

71  Cf., F. Mehrhoff & K.M. Müller, 'Klinische Sektion: erlaubt, notwendig, verboten?', *Der Pathologe*, 11 (1990), 131–36.

72  This is even done by representatives of the church, see Böckle, 'Pietät oder Nächstenliebe', 1–2.

73  For the history of informed consent see Ruth R. Faden & T.L. Beauchamp, *A History and Theory of Informed Consent* (New York, 1986).

74  This view is held even by pathologists: Mehrhoff & Müller, 'Klinische Sektion', 136.

75  'Im praktischen Leben wird es immer darauf ankommen, die Interessen der Wissenschaft und die Gefühle der Angehörigen in Einklang zu bringen'; see 'Leichensektionen', *Ärztliches Vereinsblatt*, 55 (1928), 110.

# Vacher the Ripper and the Construction of the Nineteenth-Century Sadist

## Angus McLaren

THOSE LABELLED BY nineteenth-century doctors as sex perverts – the exhibitionists, voyeurs, masochists, inverts – were all men. Indeed one commentator grumbled that, if a man stood naked in a window and was observed by a woman he could be accused of being an exhibitionist; if a woman stood naked in a window and was observed by a man he would be regarded as a voyeur. What did the labelling and condemnation of certain forms of male sexuality signify? How did such concepts make the world more intelligible? In what ways did such concepts frame notions of 'normal' masculinity? This essay focuses on the psychiatric construction of the concept of sadism in nineteenth-century France. The 'hook' on which the discussion will hang is the 1898 trial of Vacher the Ripper, which precipitated an extended discussion of sadism. The working premise is that the classification and definition of sexual pathologies by doctors represented in part a new medicalisation of sexuality. But sexology did not simply create its subjects. Sadism was as much a literary as a scientific construct. De Sade was himself a writer of fiction, many of whose themes were taken up by the decadents from the 1880s onward. If the term 'sadism' was increasingly employed by public commentators at the end of the century that did not mean that there was any necessary increase in violent sexual acts nor any real growth in psychiatric knowledge. The apparent explanatory powers of sadism, it will be suggested, were more directly related to the social and cultural pressures *fin-de-siècle* France was experiencing.

On 1 September 1895 at Bénonces (Ain) eleven-year-old Alexandre Leger was asked by a stranger to come into the woods to see something pretty. The boy refused. Later that day fifteen-year-old Jean-Marie Robin, noticing that the cattle had been allowed to wander into a clover field, set out to look for the village shepherd, sixteen-year-old Victor Portalier. Jean-Marie discovered in a ditch Victor's sexually abused, butchered, and disembowelled body. Two years later, on the afternoon of 4 August 1897, a stonecutter at Champuis (Rhône), responding to repeated cries for help, subdued and held for the gendarmes a lout who had attempted to molest a farm woman. The assailant, a vagrant by the name of Joseph Vacher, was on 7 September found guilty of assault and sentenced to three months in jail. As his description matched that of the suspected murderer of Victor Portalier, he was handed over to Émile Fourquet, a *juge d'instruction* (examining magistrate), who had since 1895 been struck by the similarity of the description of the suspects in a number of rural murders with that of the tramp seen with Portalier. Vacher was quickly identified by witnesses to the outrage at Bénonces. But to the horror of his interrogators Vacher also confessed to not only killing Portalier, but also to the murder and sexual violation of an additional seven females and four males.[1] Shouting, 'Glory to Jesus! Glory to Joan of Arc! To the greatest martyr of all time! And glory to the Great Saviour!', Joseph Vacher on 26 October 1898 entered the *cour d'assises* (Assize Court) of the department of the Ain sitting at Bourg to face the charge of murder.[2]

The question the court dealt with was not if Vacher had committed murder, but why. What sort of person was he? Vacher's simple response was that he was a madman. A multitude of witnesses concurred that Vacher had, in a brief twenty-nine years, lived a tragic and violent life. Born on 16 November 1869 at Beaufort (Isère), he came from a poor family of eleven brothers and sisters. The boy's peculiar nature was noted early on. If he cried like a dog, Vacher repeatedly insisted, it was because of the bite he had received as a child from a rabid animal. But some neighbours claimed that he had from the first been a brutal, violent and crafty character. Many of Vacher's difficulties with others were attributed to the sexual conflicts he experienced in dealing with males. He did learn to read and write and at eighteen had entered the monastery of the frères Maristes as a postulant. He left two years later. Witnesses stated that he was expelled by the brothers because he subjected some of his comrades to odious and infamous acts. At the very least he had shown 'his celery' to others and, according to a friend, 'il avait masturbé ses camarades' (he had masturbated his schoolmates) and attempted an act 'contre nature' ('unnatural' act) with twelve-year-old Marcelin Bourde.[3] On a later occasion, he attempted to climb into bed with a man whose room he was sharing. The latter reported he had threatened Vacher with a chair adding 'that we were not in Africa.'[4] Contracting a venereal disease he sought cures in Lyon where he took up the trade of papermaker. Here he again manifested an abnormally violent temper, reportedly menacing a fellow worker with a knife. Ex-employers claimed that he spouted anarchist ideas and a colleague recalled that, 'we used to say that he had a screw loose.'[5] In November 1890 Vacher began his military service at Besançon with the 60th artillery regiment. Plunged once more into an all-male environment Vacher found that his 'inversion tendencies' elicited his comrades' hostility. Unlike them he did not drink or go to the brothels. His mess mates regarded him as a bigot and brown-noser. As a 'blue' or rookie he was subjected accordingly to much rough 'hazing' that reached such levels that even his officers protested. Vacher's response, true to form, was more deadly; on one occasion he replied to the barrack room bullies' attempt to trip him up by firing his rifle at them. His fellow recruits became so terrified of the one whom they called the 'bear' or the 'madman' that they slept with bayonets unsheathed. Captain Greilsammer, Vacher's lieutenant when he was in the 60th regiment, later recalled having to report him as a bad character who was always looking for victims.

But Vacher was as much a menace to himself. He was known to cry out in his sleep and strike his head against the barrack walls and, on one occasion, tried to cut his own throat. In 1893 his incoherence was such that he was first hospitalised and then allowed to go on convalescent leave. In this confused state Vacher found himself not only taunted by men but rejected by a woman. At Beau-les-Dames he asked Louise Barrant, whom he had met in Besançon, to marry him. For the short time that he had known her he had proven himself insanely jealous of rivals, threatening her and others with a knife. When she refused his offer of marriage he shot her and then turned the gun on himself. She was slightly wounded and Vacher only succeeded in lodging a bullet in his own skull. The slug, which could not be removed from his right ear, caused deafness and facial paralysis. The attack was treated by the authorities as a simple 'crime passionnel' (crime of passion) and in July 1893 Vacher was sent to the asylum at Dole from which he reportedly twice escaped. He was arrested in Besançon, judged by the authorities to be irresponsible and sent to the asylum of St Robert in his home department. There he was treated by Dr Dufour who, after a mere five months, optimistically declared Vacher, who still had a bullet lodged in his skull, to have been restored to mental health. He was released in April 1894 and then began, in Vacher's words, his horrible 'pilgrimage', which in three years resulted in the loss of at least eleven lives.

In court the overarching argument of Vacher's melodramatic defence was that he was only responsible to God, of whom he was an instrument. He was happy to be photographed with his bible and staff on which he had inscribed words of praise for Mary of Lourdes. Raising his voice to a shout he concluded his court address with the words: 'To be able to resist my particular passion for so long required Providence to keep special watch over me.'[6] Vacher's second tack was to claim that as a child he had been bitten by a rabid dog and his blood poisoned by the medicine he was later given. The 'guilty' were therefore the empirics who sold cures for rabies. Having a bullet in his head due to his attempted suicide he described as a third extenuating circumstance. And, finally, Vacher accused Dr Dufour of the asylum of St Robert for incompetently letting loose a dangerous man. Why had so much blood been shed? The asylum doctors were guilty: 'Because of the faults of the asylums which succeeded in having the innocent turn on each other, alas.'[7] Indeed, Vacher went on to present his crimes as a sort of providential mission against psychiatry. Why had murders been committed? 'In order to provide a warning of what happens in the lunatic asylums.'[8] He compared himself to Joan of Arc, 'une martyre comme moi' (a martyr like me). 'Yes, in reading a book, I understood my mission; Joan of Arc is like me; she was locked up in an iron cage; she had to defend herself against the doctors.'[9] And Joan like him – and his victims – had been a shepherd. Vacher never denied any of his crimes; his basic argument was that none was premeditated. He insisted that the doctors who claimed he was sane were liars. How did they know what he felt or thought? He invoked the very number of his attacks as the final confirmation of his self-proclaimed madness: 'Do you believe that a man who did what I did is not mad? To say that I am responsible, is to be more criminal than me.'[10] But the court was not impressed by Vacher's railings. The accused, warned the judge, had to give up his meandering arguments and decide whether his dog bite or his providential mission were responsible for his deeds. The medical experts declared him to be sane. In the end he was found guilty and on 31 December 1898 on the Champs de Mars at Bourg before an immense clamorous crowd which bayed for his blood, he was publicly guillotined.

It might have been expected that the doctors would have been receptive to Vacher's claims to be a madman. A good deal has been written recently about the ways in which psychiatrists in late nineteenth-century trials, for both humanitarian reasons and in order to exalt their profession's expertise, advanced the concept of mental irresponsibility.[11] But in 1898 the leading French psychiatrists chose, despite all the evidence to the contrary, to regard Vacher as sane. This reflected, in part, that in the criminological world of the 1890s the Italian stress on biological determinism was being usurped by the French focus on pathological social forces.[12] Nevertheless, the medical witnesses' stance in the Vacher trial was still rather curious inasmuch as psychiatrists were saying that a man who had been twice institutionalised and who, after the repeated assaults in his regiment and the events of Baume-les-Dames was described by doctors as crazy, was actually sane. The three medical experts called by the court insisted that Vacher was neither an epileptic nor an 'impulsif' (impulsive character) but an 'immoral violent' (violent immoralist) occasionally plagued by melancholy, delirium, paranoia and thoughts of suicide. What made the diagnosis of Vacher's mental state all the more important was that it was chiefly established by France's leading expert in criminology, Professor Alexandre Lacassagne. Lacassagne is best known today as the leader of late nineteenth-century French legal medicine who fought against Cesare Lombroso and the positivist school of criminal anthropology which held that treatment rather than punishment was needed for the 'born criminals' who could not help themselves.[13] Lacassagne, a staunch defender of the death penalty, sought to shift the emphasis in criminal psychiatry from the biological to the social determinants of crime. Two of his epigrams were to become famous: 'The social milieu is the mother culture of criminality; the microbe is the criminal, an element which gains significance only at the moment when it finds the broth which makes it ferment' and 'Societies have the criminals they deserve.'[14] The French school attributed most criminal behaviour to pathological social influences such as poverty, alcoholism, poor housing, and bad companions. They advanced a positivistic message, but one sufficiently close to jurists' orthodox stress on individual responsibility to be welcomed by the courts.[15]

Lacassagne followed such a tack in the Vacher case. While Vacher screamed that the doctors were lying Lacassagne argued that the accused was sane, that he had always been playing a role and was in fact a rather maladroit simulator. To make his case Lacassagne asserted that Vacher had a 'system'. Vacher had told some witnesses, including a 'mouton' (stool pigeon or informer) placed in his cell that he only played the fool to get around the doctors. Realising early on that he might pass as a madman, he admitted only to crimes that appeared to be motiveless and claimed to act without thinking. But in fact, Lacassagne argued, proof that Vacher was not pushed solely by perverted sexual passions was indicated by evidence that he took precautions rationally, hid his bodies, robbed his victims, and successfully

eluded capture. Though offering no evidence Lacassagne further asserted
that Vacher worked with a band of 'chemineaux' (tramps) and attributed to
him up to twenty-eight other murders. And finally, Lacassagne asked how
Vacher could claim to be mad when he had been promoted by the army to
the rank of sergeant?[16] Here Lacassagne blundered; no military witnesses
imagined that madness might disqualify one from promotion.

The question of whether Vacher was insane or not cannot be
answered here. What we can attempt to trace are the social, cultural and
political preoccupations that coloured the findings of Lacassagne and his
followers. In the first place professional solidarity no doubt played a role in
the doctors' refutation of Vacher's claim to be mad. Vacher had been
declared sane by an esteemed colleague, Dr Dufour of the asylum at St
Robert. Vacher was arguing now that the psychiatrists, in releasing a
madman, were responsible for his atrocious deeds. The experts may have felt
some minor embarrassment in noting that the military doctors had been
wrong in thinking Vacher crazy, but the psychiatrists saw that to support the
accused's claim that he was insane would put them in the impossible position
of attacking their own profession and admitting to being accomplices to
murder. Drs Lacassagne, Rebatel, and Pierret accordingly concurred that
Vacher was not mad; he only pretended to be. The second motive that the
French professors of legal medicine had in demolishing Vacher's claim was
that in doing so they could demonstrate how sophisticated the science of
criminology had become. Anthropometric measurements were taken of all of
Vacher's limbs; his scars, weight, height, and eye colouring were noted and a
radiographic analysis made of his head. Investigations were carried out to
determine that he bore no signs of physical degeneration, that he suffered
from no debilitating childhood sickness, that his family contained no mad,
epileptic or idiotic members. The experts conceded that the bullet in
Vacher's head – the wound still suppurating – did cause facial paralysis on the
right side of his face and deafness in one ear, but cheerfully noted that
Vacher had no history of hallucinations.[17] Thanks to the autopsy carried out
after Vacher's execution the voyeuristic public further learnt that he had a
large penis and an atrophied left testicle, but a normal anus and, therefore,
had not been a passive pederast. His brain, which weighed 1500 grams, was
sliced open by the doctors who declared it to be normal. It was photographed
and a mould taken of it. No one found it ironic that the medical experts, who
condemned Vacher for mutilating his victims, proceeded after his execution
to subject his body to such a meticulous dissection.[18] In short, all the sorts of
efforts made by criminal anthropologists – in particular the Italians – to
detect the stigmata of the born criminal were made and the findings declared

by the French to be of no great importance. Lacassagne authoritatively asserted that those who might claim that a bloodthirsty killer like Vacher would have to have been suffering from some major physical or psychological handicap were proved wrong; there was nothing irresistible or impulsive in Vacher's acts. The third and, for the purposes of this essay, most important preoccupation which coloured Lacassagne's view of the Vacher case was the interest in the new concept of sadism. Vacher's trial was not responsible for spawning the concept, but it provided the occasion for nineteenth-century French psychiatrists' most extensive discussion of the term. Why did Vacher commit his bloody deeds? Lacassagne quoted extensively from the psychiatric report on Menesclou, the 1880 murderer, which helpfully contrasted 'imbéciles de l'intelligence' (the mentally deficient) with 'débiles du sentiment' (moral imbeciles). The latter, though reasoning beings, claimed Lacassagne, did not have the moral repugnances of the normal. Vacher manifested just such failings by his dabbling in anarchism, vagabondism, and homosexuality.[19] Lacassagne's point was that Vacher was not insane, but an antisocial sadist. His acts were the work of a 'monstrous criminal', not those of a madman.[20] And as horrific as sadists might be, many were completely sane. Vacher was a sadist who was aroused by the sight of flesh, but that did not make him irresponsible.[21]

What did Lacassagne mean by sadism? Dr Marciat, who contributed a discussion of sadism to Lacassagne's volume on Vacher began with Thoinot's definition.[22] 'The perversion of the genital instinct, that is known today, by the name of sadism consists in finding suffering in a human being a condition always necessary and at times sufficient for sexual enjoyment; this suffering is of a very variable degree,—at times slight, at times severe or of a degree of atrocious refinement,—and the subject either causes it to be inflicted, or sees it inflicted, or finally inflicts it himself on some human being.'[23] Yet what sadism was from the point of view of legal medicine was left rather vague; no specific act was required. Lacassagne and his colleagues used the term as a sort of moral label to designate those who were monsters but not mad. The term 'sadism' had first been used on rare occasions by critics in the 1850s to describe the decadent themes found in the writings of Flaubert and Baudelaire.[24] The word only began to be widely employed in the 1880s. De Sade, who had been almost forgotten for much of the nineteenth century, was simultaneously rediscovered in the 1880s by both psychiatrists and novelists. Isidore Liseux republished *Justine*, *Juliette*, and *La philosophie dans le boudoir*, and several biographies of the marquis soon followed.[25] Few may have actually read de Sade's works very closely, but an interest in his ideas quickly mushroomed. They drew the attention in

England of Swinburne and of Wilde and in Germany of Herbst, Eulenberg, Rutter and of Blaubert, but his first and greatest appeal was in France.[26] Those decadents who dabbled in sadistic themes of black masses, the occult, demonic pederasty, and flagellation, who declared self-conscious evil better than ignorance, and who envisaged society culminating in sacrifice and death, included the Goncourts, Guillaume Apollinaire, Barbey d'Aurevilly, Léon Bloy, Paul Bourget, Villiers de l'Isle-Adam, Rachilde (Marguerite Eymery), J.K. Huysmans, Jean Lorraine, and Pierre Louys.[27] Most of the literary acolytes of de Sade, though they paraded their irreverence and atheism, were on the political right, avowed enemies of mass society. Fictional and medical portrayals of sadism fed off each other. Lacassagne noted Dostoievski's remarks on the well known correlation between beatings and sexual arousal and went on to say that Zola's *La Bête humaine* – inspired by accounts of Jack the Ripper's murders – was 'a wonderful confirmation of the notion of the relations which link sex and violence.'[28] Alfred Binet similarly drew many of his references to fetishes from fiction. And the sexually troubled learnt to be as much influenced by literature as were doctors. Serge Paul reported that patients by the 1890s were already citing in their defence the works of de Sade, Jean-Jacques Rousseau, and Sacher-Masoch.[29] The literary notion of sadism popularised in the 1880s and 1890s was primarily a manifestation of an elitist disdain for the conventions of middle-class and mass society. The perverse was personified by libertarian noblemen like Gilles de Rais, de Sade and Des Esseintes. But, ironically the real men of the *fin de siècle* whose actual acts led psychiatrists to label them as sadists were for the most part, like Vacher, crude and violent members of the very lower classes whom the decadent novelists most feared. The 'real' sadists, far from being powerful, sexual supermen, were slaves to their own compulsive behaviour.[30]

When turning from the literary world to the sexological writings of the late nineteenth century much is discovered of the same morbid fascination with perversions. The tabloids, police files, decadent novels and psychiatric journals shared similar vocabularies and concerns. The European presses churned out popular bestiaries of sadists or lust murderers, both the medical accounts and literary chronicles of behavioural aberrations producing the same sort of fetishistic literature that blended biography and clinical case histories of exemplary perverts.[31] The work of one of Lacassagne's colleagues, Dr Alexis Lepaulard's *Vampirisme: nécrophilie, nécrosadisme, nécrophage* (Lyon, 1901), was a typical compilation. Such medical studies contained much moralising and little analysis. Their authors usually adopted a scatter-gun approach, beginning with Gilles de Rais, the fourteenth-century killer of children, and then hopping three centuries to the marquis de Sade himself. For the nineteenth century they could be counted on to include Leger, Menesclou, Jack the Ripper, and a host of lesser villains.[32] What sorts of threats precipitated the construction of sadism? It might be imagined that the sadist represented the danger posed by a hypermasculinity. Certainly the creation of the concept of 'sadism' spoke to a contemporary concern for gender relations. Sadism, like all the perversions catalogued in the late nineteenth century, was a gendered notion which could only be fully understood in the context of what contemporaries saw as appropriate male or female behaviour; that men were supposed to be aggressive and women passive.[33] Aggressiveness had both its costs and benefits. Because males were supposed to be the sexually aggressive and adventurous sex, doctors assumed that only males could be perverts. As the male was more cerebral than the female his mind was more likely to overcome his body. His desires could be degraded, and decline from the active to the passive, from the genital to the oral, from the masculine to the effeminate. Much if not all homosexuality, for example, was said to result from sexual excesses and exhaustion.[34] Impotency was presented by physicians like Tardieu as the revenge of the body which had given way to deviant desires. Nineteenth-century experts now presented a variety of corrupt practices – including masturbation and sodomy – which were once seen as choices, as symptoms of the entire personality of dangerous 'others'. Doctors disciplined other men in inventing and brandishing such labels as masochist, exhibitionist, and sadist; what previously had been regarded as momentary sexual preferences were increasingly taken as revelations of the whole of a person's being.[35] Doctors claimed that females, despite evidence to the contrary, were largely inhibited by their innate passivity from actively indulging in such vices. Alfred Binet's famous account of the fetishes accordingly described only men's fixations on lips, hair, hands and boots.[36] Given the general assumption of sexual asymmetry it followed that Binet took a man's being attracted to an old, ugly woman as an indication of some fetishistic appeal, while he found nothing puzzling about a young woman's marriage to an old, ugly man. Money, despite what Marx had said, was not regarded by doctors as a fetish. Sadism has to be understood as just such a gendered perversion which French doctors employed for both descriptive and prescriptive purposes. Richard von Krafft-Ebing, the German sexologist, has often been credited with coining the term, but as he himself made clear it was already being employed in France when *Psychopathia Sexualis* appeared in 1886 and his boast was simply that he coined, as sadism's analogue, the concept of 'masochism'.[37] Doctors, in speaking of 'sadism', were taking over a concept popularised by writers of fiction and accordingly an historical analysis of the concept has to take into account why, in the cultural context of the 1880s and 1890s, such an idea was 'good to think with.'[38]

How did doctors employ the concept? Sadism was first turned to by sexologists not to curb but to incite male aggressiveness. Krafft-Ebing, whom Lacassagne frequently cited, stated there were wide gradations of sadism. At the most innocent level stood the husband who, in asking for sex in unusual locales or in employing force in the conjugal act, exhibited sadistic tendencies. 'It seems probable that this sadistic force is developed by the natural shyness and modesty of woman towards the aggressive manners of the male, especially during the earlier periods of married life and particularly when the husband is hypersexual. Woman no doubt derives pleasure from her innate coyness and the final victory of the man affords her intense and refined gratification. Hence the frequent recurrence of these little love comedies.'[39] The atavistic notion – that in times past sex followed assault – was carried on by the aptly named André Lamoureux who saw sadism as an hereditary trait of the male seizing the female.[40] Such atavisms resurfaced occasionally. Krafft-Ebing cited the case of a man who could only make love to his wife after having made himself angry, and Moll that of a boy who could only get an erection when resisted.[41] Even in 'normal' sexual relations sexologists detected in the desire to tease or mock a loved one a remnant of cruelty. In England, Havelock Ellis in his discussion of 'Love and Pain' followed the same line in presenting wooing as a domesticated form of the earlier violent male pursuit of the female. Males delighted in displaying force and in the 'simulacrum of pain', their 'arousal' depended on a degree of female resistance. Women delighted in submitting and as they had to be penetrated the ideas of pain and pleasure were necessarily mingled in the female mind. Accordingly, there existed a biological justification for a degree of male sexual violence.[42] Normal men had an impulse to give pain and normal women an impulse to receive it: 'So that we need not unduly deprecate the 'cruelty' of men within these limits, nor unduly commiserate the women who are subjected to it.'[43] In other words, a normal man was in a sense 'naturally' sadistic and a normal woman 'naturally' masochistic. At the same time, doctors were warning their male readers that masculinity was not the fundamental and unalterable element they might have imagined, but rather something fragile. Without a conscious effort of the will to spurn vice it was possible potentially to spin off into the perversions.[44] Some, like Dimitry Stefanowsky in an 1892 article in the *Archives d'anthropologie criminelle*, confusingly spoke of male 'sadistic passivity', what Krafft-Ebing more clearly called masochism. But all commentators agreed that masochism, being an inherent female trait, was only a 'true perversion' in a man; commentators specifically defined the syndrome as the sexual pleasure a man associated with the idea of being humiliated by a woman. The vice, according to Laurent, was a manifestation of a male's abdication of his legitimate domination.[45] For French readers the most famous description of a youth's discovery of his masochistic feelings was that which Rousseau confided to his *Confessions*. 'To be on my knees before an imperious mistress, to obey her orders, to have to ask her forgiveness, were for me the sweetest pleasures; the more my lively imagination inflamed my blood, the more I felt like an overwhelmed lover.'[46] Stefanowsky described the man who gave oral sex to a woman as a passivist who was subjecting himself to a 'femme sadiste' (sadistic woman). Such passivity, if unchecked, could lead on to the victim's sexual inversion and the ultimate degradation – that of becoming a fellator of other men.

The pervasive misogyny of the 1890s manifested itself in numerous literary and artistic portrayals of feminine evil in the guises of the invalid, vamp or vampire. Novelists like Mirbeau were fixated on the notion of the sadistic woman. Though the sexologists regarded sadism as primarily a male perversion they dutifully noted that cruel, 'masculine' women like Salome, Messalina and Catherine de Médici warranted the titles of illustrious female sadists. Dr Erich Wulffen, a German expert in legal medicine, labelled as sadistic such French women as Rose Lacombe, Théroigne de Méricourt and Louise Michel who, by participating in radical politics, had violated gender boundaries.[47] If men had a sadistic streak, women's masochism was, doctors agreed, so natural as not to count as a perversion. Thus, they followed the old idea posited by Michelet and Comte that woman were more 'alive to the chain of self-sacrifice.'[48] Indeed, Serge Paul noted that since a woman was meant to serve it was hard to notice a masochistic female. In Russia, he claimed, the blows a woman received were taken as proof of her spouse's love.[49] In America, it was believed, wrote G. Stanley Hall in his classic text on adolescence, that there was something wrong with the young man who was not aggressive.[50] In short, the concept of 'sadism' was first employed by doctors to foster certain forms of male sexuality. They, like many other late nineteenth-century commentators, believed that civilised men were most threatened, not by excess passion, but by the enervation spawned by urban life.

Sadism's second function was to censor certain forms of sexual behaviour. Although the sexologists told men that they were supposed to be sexually aggressive, there were limits. According to Binet the line between healthy sexual excitation and perversion was crossed when the fetishistic act became more important than the heterosexual intercourse to which it was supposed to lead. When the pain inflicted became the chief source of a man's sexual pleasure he became a pervert. Exactly the same practice, if it abetted heterosexual intercourse, could be deemed healthy. Doctors described the lust murder of the sadist not as an act which could be located at the aggressive extreme on the continuum of normal male violence, but as an aberrant crime that had nothing to do with heterosexuality. Healthy masculinity emerged unscathed if not reinvigorated from such analyses which began with the premise that sex crimes were individual deviant acts, not distorted reflections of normal gender relations. In creating the 'sadist' doctors constructed a creature who roamed somewhere beyond the norms of masculine sexual aggressiveness.

Was sadism a result of unleashed primitive passions or the product of overrefinement; a sign of hypermasculinity or an evidence of effeminacy and impotency? The most serious version of sadism – lust murder – Krafft-Ebing designated a 'primitive anomaly'. 'It is a disturbance (a deviation) in the evolution of psychosexual processes sprouting from the soil of psychical degeneration.'[51] Males, needing to win and conquer women, were necessarily aggressive but under pathological conditions such a drive could 'likewise be excessively developed, and express itself in an impulse to subdue absolutely the object of desire, even to destroy or kill it.'[52] Lust awakened cruelty and cruelty awakened lust. Lust and anger were often linked and in the abnormal the customary inhibitory checks were absent. Yet, some in whom the sadistic instinct existed from birth managed, according to Krafft-Ebing, to fight off such urges. In France the more common view was that perversions were not simply inherited but acquired as a result of being overcivilised. According to Serge Paul and Valentin Magnan civilisation needed boundaries.[53] But the luxurious, feverish life of the city led to excesses, alcoholism, menstrual problems, tuberculosis, and psychiatric troubles. Sexual perversions followed. Once their senses were jaded, the blasé turned to sadism.[54] Krafft-Ebing declared sadism to be congenital; the French, though they conceded that the degenerate were particularly susceptible, asserted it to be an acquired vice. Sadism accordingly was presented by French psychiatrists as a product of insufficient rather than excessive masculinity. Lacassagne envisaged the brain having special organs which presided over the functioning of the two instincts of reproduction and destruction. The genital instinct was, aside from the instinct for self-preservation, the strongest and should normally predominate. Signs of effeminacy or homosexuality provided evidence that the reproductive drive was incapacitated; if that happened the instinct for destruction could take over and sadism result.

The third way in which doctors employed the concept of sadism was to alert the public to the dangers of a male manifesting feminine traits. To understand why a man's effeminacy would be considered dangerous it has to be remembered that nineteenth-century medical scientists were in the process of drawing a sharp line between what were called the 'opposite' sexes. The fact of sexual incommensurability and the demands of reproduction, they asserted, governed all aspects of life and any blurring of the gender roles smacked of the perverse. Accordingly, the term 'féminisme' first came into common usage in France about the same time as the term 'sadisme' and for related reasons. 'Féminisme' was originally used by doctors in the 1870s in the pathological sense to describe the physical and psychological ways in which a man might manifest certain female characteristics.[55] Pierre Garnier, for example, referred to homosexuality and neurasthenia as being engendered by a man's feminism. Charles Féré asserted that feminine characteristics (féminisme, gynécomstie) were manifested by the man who suffered the 'sexual death' of losing his genitals.[56] Women writers were only to appropriate the term and employ it in a positive sense from the 1890s onward. Doctors who employed 'féminisme' in the pathological sense were not so much attacking the 'nouvelle femme' as the possibility of the emergence of a 'nouvel homme'. Both sadism and feminism, they asserted, were manifestations of a dangerous lack of virility. Lacassagne argued that the sexual passions of the sadist were not masculine but essentially feminine. According to his captors, Vacher was always in search of flesh, was always like a woman in rut. 'The sadist,' declared Lacassagne, 'has something of the cerebral licentiousness of the woman.'[57] Such assertions linked up with the old idea that the woman was preoccupied by sex all the time; the normal man only occasionally.

The fourth function of the concept of sadism was its use by medical men as a stick with which to beat back the threat of inversion (as homosexuality was called in the late nineteenth century). If normal women were preoccupied by sex all the time, so too, according to the psychiatrists, were some abnormal men – homosexuals. Accordingly, at Vacher's trial great stress was placed on the accused's inversion tendencies. Fourquet, the investigating magistrate, expressed surprise that Vacher, who among his fellow tramps had the reputation of being a pederast, should have wooed Louise Barrant. 'Until his arrival in the army, Vacher appeared to have never been attracted to any woman. No romantic adventures were found in his past. Besides, he was a pederast and no one had ever noticed him looking for women until his induction into the 60th artillery regiment.'[58] Lacassagne, in describing Vacher's murdering and sodomising of Pierre Massot-Pellet,

Victor Portalier, and the shepherds at Courzieu and Tassin-La Demi Lune, concluded that these young herdsman inflamed Vacher with a lubricious passion. When women in the audience expressed their shock at hearing such accounts the judge took obvious pleasure in retorting, 'Too bad for you ladies, you were warned; you should not be here.'[59] The doctor, in further reporting that in one of the interrogations Vacher admitted that young men had a power of attraction over him, concluded: 'Yes, there is the truth; Vacher had always been a pederast, later he became a murderer and sadist.'[60] Such linkages were even made by those who tried to avoid tarring all homosexuals with the same brush. André Raffalovich, for example, asserted that in Europe sodomy was the delight of only 'the ignorant, the violent, the criminal, the cruel, the masochistic, the sadistic.'[61] The term homosexual, coined in 1869 by the Swiss doctor Karoly Maria Benkert, was not to displace the term 'invert' until the twentieth century. Lacassagne, in an earlier study devoted to pederasty, had followed Brouardel and Tardieu in attributing 'sexual inversion' to a poorly balanced nervous system marked by infantilism and lack of masculine energy.[62] Some were 'native' or congenital homosexuals; others drifted into the vice as a result of impotence, onanism or a fear of women. Whether or not homosexuality was innate or acquired Lacassagne insisted on referring to it as a 'school for crime' and listed a string of murders with which the perversion was associated. Henri Joly and Benjamin Ball provided similar lurid accounts of the dangers posed by perverts who raped and killed children.[63] Octave Uzanne noted with some surprise that by 1900 the notion of sadism, which fifteen years previously had only been of interest to the advanced literary set, had become a central preoccupation of those who studied male prostitution and sexual inversion.[64]

The purpose of this investigation was to determine how and why the concept of sadism was first employed. What has been found is that it was used not to describe simply the deviant, but to shore up certain preconceived notions of manliness. The question remains why such concerns were so strongly felt. Why were French doctors preoccupied by male sexual deviancy? Why did the press, at the turn of the century, assert that the family was threatened and traditional gender roles under attack? One answer is that the French, with the lowest birth rate in nineteenth-century Europe, were particularly preoccupied by the notion of incapacitated reproductive drives. From 1850 onwards biological fears of degeneration were extended by alarmists to explain both family and social problems. After France's defeat by Germany in 1870 a full-blown depopulation hysteria developed, only to be followed in neighbouring countries in the 1890s. There, too, the mood of sombre despair deepened in the century's last decades as doctors brandished the threats that drugs, alcohol, and syphilis posed the family. The fall in fertility – attributed to short-sighted egoism – and the pro-natalist rhetoric to which it gave rise played a central role in the 'discovery' in France of male sexual perversions. The nation's sense of guilt, precipitated by the drop in the birth rate, obviously led to the hunt for scapegoats on whom anxieties could be projected. Psychiatry exploited such fears; although the science was perceived by many as being anticlerical, if anything it outstripped the Catholic church in its condemnations of the moral egoism that was supposedly weakening the nation. Thus, for example, Étienne Martin, professor of legal medicine at Lyon, attributed Vacher's sadism to the fact that as an isolated individual he had no natural curb on his insatiable needs. The normal man had the 'duties and charms of family' to act as brake on his sex drive, but rules of love were missing for the violent and brutal. Vacher's sadistic assaults, the doctors warned, represented merely the ultimate manifestation of unbridled egoism.[65] Gabriel Tarde, the conservative jurist and crowd psychologist known for his development of the concept of criminal suggestion, followed a similar line in the chapter he contributed to Lacassagne's volume on Vacher. Tarde pessimistically argued that advances of civilisation led to increases in criminality. In particular, he held the press responsible for exploiting sensational crime stories and so contributing to a contagion of murder, blackmail, and pornography.[66] The fall in fertility rates he attributed also to the force of 'imitation'.[67] What the rise of the new, nervous, suggestible society represented, in his eyes, was the decline of the patriarchal family with its 'serenity' and 'majestic particularism'. Given the intemperance and temptations *fin-de-siècle* society dangled before free-floating individuals, killing did not have to be attributed to the peculiarities of the 'born' criminal. All men were placed at risk and only the strong could resist. 'The psychology of the murderer,' Tarde declared gloomily, 'is the psychology of everybody.'[68]

Sadism was a versatile concept that could be turned to a variety of purposes. In the literary world novelists, who remained true to the stalest misogynistic clichés, used it to parade a fresh irreverence. In the psychiatric world its discussion began with what appeared to be a critique of masculinity, but concluded with its defence. Sexual aggressiveness was part of the normal masculine psyche; only when pushed beyond the limits of the 'normal' was it described by doctors as a sign of impotency rather than potency, of femininity rather than of masculinity. More sharply demarcated notions of active masculinity and passive femininity accordingly emerged from the first discussions of sadism. The new biomedical models of masculinity and femininity served ideological functions. Doctors claimed that it was 'natural' or a 'timeless' practice for men to use force to subdue females, yet it is known that the notion of the passionless female was, in fact, a new nineteenth-century creation. Traditionally women were seen to be as much interested in sex as males and indeed as potentially insatiable. Late nineteenth-century doctors, in advancing complementary psychological models of the aggressive male and the passive female, were responding to a demand. There existed a reading public that wanted to be reassured that despite the host of social changes which appeared to blur gender divisions, deep psychic cleavages necessarily separated the sexes. In locating the emergence of the concept of sadism in the context of this reordering of gender roles it becomes clear that doctors were reflecting society's belief that the threats modern life posed the virility of the mass of ordinary men was far more worrying than the violence of the isolated pervert.[69]

*The permission of The University of Chicago Press is gratefully acknowledged for the materials contained in this essay which constitutes portions of one chapter in Angus McLaren's* Trials of Masculinity: Policing Sexual Boundaries, 1870–1930 *(Chicago, 1997 & 1999).*

# Notes

1 M. Laurent-Martin, *Le Roi des assassins* (Paris, 1897); Emile Fourquet, *Vacher* (Paris, 1931).

2 *Gazette de Tribunaux*, 27 October 1898, p. 987.

3 Alexandre Lacassagne, 'Vacher l'Eventreur', *Archives de l'anthropologie criminelle* 13 (1898), 641.

4 Fourquet, *Vacher*, p. 235.

5 Lacassagne, 'Vacher', 641.

6 *Gazette de Tribunaux*, 31 October–1 November 1898, p. 1004.

7 Ibid., p. 1004.

8 Ibid., p. 1004.

9 Ibid., p. 1004.

10 Ibid., p. 1004.

11 Ruth Harris, *Murders and Madness: Medicine, Law, and Society in the Fin-de-Siècle* (Oxford, 1989); Jan Goldstein, *Console and Classify: The French Psychiatric Profession in the Nineteenth Century* (Cambridge, 1987); Robert A. Nye, *Crime, Madness and Politics in Modern France: The Medical Concept of National Decline* (Princeton, 1984), Patrizia Guarnieri, *A Case of Child Murder: Law and Science in Nineteenth-Century Tuscany* (Cambridge, 1993).

12 Ian R. Dowbiggin, *Inheriting Madness: Professionalization and Psychiatric Knowledge in Nineteenth-Century France* (Berkeley, 1991).

13 Émile Laurent, *L'Anthropologie criminelle et les nouvelles théories du crime* (Paris, 1893).

14 See Robert Nye, 'Heredity or Milieu: The Foundations of Modern European Criminological Theory', *Isis*, 67 (1976), 339; Nye, *Madness*, pp. 103–6, 191–92, 221–24.

15 See Alexandre Berard, *La responsibilité morale* (Lyon, 1892).

16 Alexandre Lacassagne, *Vacher l'Éventreur et les crimes sadiques* (Lyon, 1899) p. 286.

17 Lacassagne, *Vacher*, pp. 57–59.

18 Édouard Toulouse, *Le Rapport des médicins expert sur Vacher* (Clermont, 1898); Alexandre Lacassagne, 'Le cerveau de Vacher', *Archives de l'anthropologie criminelle*, 14 (1899), 653–62; M.J.V. Laborde avec la collaboration de MM. Manouvrier, Papillault & Gelle, *Étude psycho-physiologique, médico-légal & anatomique sur Vacher* (Paris, 1900).

19 *Gazette de Tribunaux*, 31 October–1 November 1898, p. 1004.

20 Lacassagne, 'Vacher', 636.

21 Lacassagne, *Vacher*, p. 288.

22 Marciat, 'Le Marquis de Sade et le sadisme' in Lacassagne, *Vacher*, pp. 185–238.

23  L. Thoinot and A.W. Weysse, *Medicolegal Aspects of Moral Offenses* (Philadelphia, 1921), p. 417.

24  *Le Grand Robert de la langue française* (Paris, 1985).

25  Octave Uzanne, *Idées sur les romans, par D.A.F. Sade* (Paris, 1878); Charles Henry, *La Verité sur le marquis de Sade* (Paris, 1887), H. d'Almeras, *Le Marquis de Sade* (Paris, 1906), Guillaume Apollinaire, *L'Oeuvre du marquis de Sade* (Paris, 1909).

26  Mario Praz, *The Romantic Agony* (New York, 1970); Jean Pierrot, *The Decadent Imagination* tr. Derek Coltman (Chicago, 1981); Jennifer Birkett, *The Sins of the Fathers: Decadence in France, 1870–1914* (London, 1986).

27  Emily Apter, *Feminizing the Fetish: Psychoanalysis and Narrative Obsession in Turn-of-the-Century France* (Ithaca, 1991), p. 128; Deborah L. Silverman, *Art Nouveau in Fin-de-Siècle France* (Berkeley, 1989).

28  Lacassagne, *Vacher*, p. 276; and for similar praise, see Scipio Sighele, *Litterature et criminalité* (Paris, 1908), pp. 132–34.

29  But for the argument that the decadent writers were themselves sick, see Dr Émile Laurent, *La poésie décadente devant la science psychiatrique* (Paris, 1897).

30  Paul Garnier, 'Des Perversions sexuelles obsédantes et impulsives', *Archives de l'anthropologie criminelle*, 15 (1900), 618.

31  See Cesare Lombroso, *L'Homme criminel* (Paris, 1887); Arthur MacDonald, *Le Criminel-type dans quelques formes graves de la criminalité*, tr. Henry Coutagne (Lyon, 1894).

32  Lacassagne, *Vacher*, pp. 265–70; Dr Serge Paul, *Le Vice et l'amour* (Paris, 1905).

33  Édouard Toulouse, *Les Conflits intersexuelles et sociaux* (Paris, 1904), p. 4; Charles Féré, *Pathologie des émotions* (Paris, 1892), pp. 479–80.

34  J.M. Charcot and V. Magnan, 'Inversion du sens génital', *Archive de neurologie*, 3–4 (1882), 53–60, 296–322.

35  Robert Nye, *Masculinity and Male Codes of Honor in Modern France* (New York, 1993).

36  Alfred Binet, 'Le fetichisme dans l'amour', *Revue philosophique*, 24 (1887), 143–67; 252–77.

37  Richard von Krafft-Ebing, *Psychopathia Sexualis* tr. Franklin S. Klaf (New York, 1965), pp. 87, 417 n12. For the assertion that Krafft-Ebing coined 'sadism' see, for example, Frank J. Solloway, *Freud: Biologist of the Mind* (New York, 1979), p. 483; H.F. Ellenberger, *The Discovery of the Unconscious* (New York, 1970), p. 299.

38  The Index-Catalogue of the Library of the Surgeon General's Office did not include 'sadism' as a topic in its first series (1891), but the second (1910) listed nine books (four in German and five in French) and forty-two articles on the subject. On the use of ideas 'good to think with' in cultural history see Robert Darnton, *The Great Cat Massacre and Other Episodes in French Cultural History* (New York, 1984).

39  Krafft-Ebing, *Psychopathia Sexualis*, pp. 53–54.

40 André Lamoureux, *De l'éventration au point de vue médico-légal* (Lyon, 1891).

41 Albert Moll, *Die Kontrare Sexualempfindung* (Berlin, 1893), pp. 186–87.

42 Margaret Jackson, *The 'Real' Facts of Life: Feminism and the Politics of Sexuality 1850–1940* (London, 1994).

43 Havelock Ellis, *Studies in the Psychology of Sex* (New York, 1936), 1: 2: 104.

44 E. Gley, 'Les Aberrations de l'instinct sexuel', *Revue philosophique*, 17 (1884), 66–92.

45 Émile Laurent, *Sadisme et masochisme* (Paris, 1903).

46 Paul, *Le Vice*, p. 169.

47 *Woman as Sexual Criminal* (New York, 1934), p. 287.

48 August Comte, *System of Positive Polity* (London, 1877), 4: 100.

49 Paul, *Le Vice*, p. 146.

50 E. Anthony Rotundo, *American Manhood: Transformations from the Revolution to the Modern Era* (New York, 1993), p. 269.

51 Krafft-Ebing, *Psychopathia Sexualis*, p. 54.

52 Krafft-Ebing, *Psychopathia Sexualis*, p. 56.

53 Paul, *Le Vice*; for the argument that 'morbid love' was usually related to anatomical anomalies, see Féré, *Pathologie*, p. 434.

54 Binet, 'Fetichisme', 266.

55 *Le Grand Robert de la langue française* (Paris, 1985) notes 'féminisme' was used by Fourier (1837); and employed in a medical sense by 1877 and in a political sense by 1904.

56 Pierre Garnier, *Anomalies sexuelles: apparentes et cachées* (Paris, 1889), p. 371; Féré, *Pathologie*, p. 495; and see also Jules Dallemagne, *Théories de la criminalité* (Paris, 1896), p. 175.

57 Lacassagne, *Vacher*, p. 288.

58 Fourquet, *Vacher*, p. 80; and see also p. 242.

59 Fourquet, *Vacher*, p. 323.

60 Lacassagne, *Vacher*, p. 33.

61 André Raffalovich, 'Unisexualité anglaise', *Archives de l'anthropologie criminelle*, 11 (1896), 431.

62 Alexandre Lacassagne, 'Péderastie', *Dictionnaire encyclopédique des sciences médicales*, 2nd series (Paris, 1886), 22: 239–59; and see also Julian Chevalier, *Sur l'inversion de l'instinct sexuel au point de vue médico-légal* (Lyon, 1893).

63 Benjamin Ball, *La folie érotique* (Paris, 1888), p. 116, 147; Henri Joly, *Le Crime: étude sociale* (Paris, 1888), pp. 124–25.

64 Uzanne in Duehren, *De Sade*, p. xv; Moll noted homosexual cases of sadism as did Ulrichs who in *Incube* (1896) spoke of lovers' bites and scratches.

65  Étienne Martin, 'Vacher devant la cour d'assises de l'Ain' in Lacassagne, *Vacher*,
    p. 67.

66  Tarde, 'Les transformations de l'impunité' in Lacassagne, *Vacher*, pp. 167–84; and on
    suggestion, see also Dr Haury, 'Les faux témoins pathologiques', *Archives de
    l'anthropologie criminelle*, 27 (1912), 637–53.

67  For the argument that the rise of 'ripper' style killings was also due to imitation, see
    M.J.F.A. de St Vincent de Paroism, *Du dépecage criminel* (Lyon, 1902).

68  Gabriel Tarde, *Penal Philosophy* (Boston, 1912), p. 256; and see also Tarde, *The Laws
    of Imitation* (New York, 1903); Arsène Dumont, *Dépopulation et civilisation: étude
    démographique* (Paris, 1990 [first ed. 1890]), pp. 402–10; Susannah Barrows,
    *Distorting Mirrors: Visions of the Crowd in Late Nineteenth-Century France* (New
    Haven, 1981), pp. 137–45.

69  Annelise Mauge, *L'Identité masculine en crise au tournant du siècle, 1871–1914* (Paris,
    1987); Michèle Perrot, 'The New Eve and the Old Adam; Changes in French
    Women's Condition at the Turn of the Century' in M.R. Higonnet et al. (eds.),
    *Behind the Lines: Gender and the Two World Wars* (New Haven, 1987), pp. 51–60.

# Prosecution and Popularity: the Case of the Dutch Sequah, 1891–1893

## Willem de Blécourt

## The Scene

THE PREVAILING OPINION about medical licensing systems in Europe is that they were the most rigid in countries and regions that had been subjected to Napoleonic rule.[1] This includes the Netherlands. Although in the course of the nineteenth century licensing laws were amended twice, in 1818 and in 1865, until recently it remained illegal to practice medicine without official qualifications in the Netherlands. Licenses were granted only to those who had followed a formal medical education, at a medical school or, since 1876, exclusively at a university. Unlicensed practitioners ran the perpetual risk of being prosecuted, fined and, in cases of severe recidivism, jailed. If cognisance is also taken of the comparatively early foundation of the Dutch Society for the Repression of Quackery in 1880 (a German equivalent only came into being in 1903) the Netherlands could be depicted easily as a quack's hell. Daily practice, however, was quite different for there was a wide gap between the letter of the law and its enforcement.[2] Prosecution had never been fierce and, at the beginning of the twentieth century, the yearly average of convictions had fallen to a national total of six.[3] Rather than deterring unlicensed healers from practising, prosecution enhanced their fame. Protestant politicians, in particular, were known to support and even to consult irregular medical practitioners.

The prosecution of unlicensed healers can be seen as a defining element of medical professionalisation. Regular physicians, by accusing other healers as being unfit to practice medicine and thereby criminalising them, determined the boundaries of their own profession as well as their own social status. As Roy Porter has commented: 'Quacks are those doctors excluded from professional power and privilege'.[4] Yet, the attempt by licensed doctors to oust their competitors did not depend only on favourable laws and the co-operation of the state prosecution system; it also needed public support. This was the flaw in the application of the Medical Acts for it depended mostly on licensed practitioners not only to initiate the prosecution of their illegal counterparts but also, to be legally valid, the complaints had to be endorsed by witnesses. Public prosecutors had to be convinced that the healer to be prosecuted was not just officially registered, which was relatively easy to establish but, in addition, that his activity could be categorised as the practice of medicine. The latter was open to discussion as it could be argued that if someone had not undergone formal medical training, then what he practised was not medicine in the official sense. Furthermore, it had to be established that the suspect practised medicine regularly and as a trade rather than helping out of necessity, as was the case when a legally qualified physician was unable to attend. And these were only the legal arguments.

Other factors that hindered the implementation of the Medical Acts were associated with the prevalent cultural assumptions about health and healing and it is necessary to consider the popularity of irregular healers to discover these assumptions. Although the immediate reasons why a healer attracted patients do not have to equal the reasons why it was hard to prosecute him, the underlying motivations will have been similar for both. Since there is no systematically collected corpus of patients' documentation for illegal healers,[5] and since their patients' books have only rarely survived,[6] it is usually impossible to discover by whom, how often, from where and for what kinds of misfortune they were consulted. Other sources to determine their popularity are needed and newspaper reports are the most suitable for this purpose.[7] Even a single report can reveal details about the flow of patients that a healer attracted on a certain day, or about the medical encounter between healer and patient. A collection of newspaper accounts, moreover, may reveal the scope and the length of a healer's practice and of possible changes in them. This paper, based primarily on newspaper accounts, presents a case study of one of the most popular and famous healers in the modern Netherlands. He was known as Sequah.[8] 'When your legs are painful', the boys in the street used to sing, 'when you suffer from rheumatism, you go to Sequah: he cures you with music'.[9]

## Enters a Healer

IN JUNE 1891 an Englishman arrived in the Netherlands. He was called Charles A. Davenport and he was employed by the Sequah Company in London to sell remedies against rheumatism. The company also provided him with his public name: Sequah. 'The provinces which Sequah traversed are the most backward, in terms of education, in the enlightened kingdom of Holland' reported the English trade journal, *Chemist and Druggist*, at the end of August 1891. This was merely an attempt to belittle the activity of Davenport who, at that stage, had not proceeded beyond Roozendaal, a small town in the province of Noord-Brabant.[10] At the beginning of Davenport's stay his chances of success did not look very promising. 'I've been in Holland with little Davenport', wrote a representative of the company to the London headquarters in June. He continued: 'I don't think it will be a big do there as cases are hard to get – it may get better further up the country'.[11] The initial failure to attract sufferers had more to do with public scepticism than with Davenport's public persona. People waited for results before they submitted themselves to his treatment. A report from a local newspaper in Roozendaal shows this quite clearly, even though it relied, in part, on Davenport's own publicity material:

> A few days ago an English doctor by the name of Sequah arrived here. With the aid of the so-called Indian prairie flower and Sequah oil the doctor tries to heal bad or malfunctioning indigestion, illness of the liver, rheumatism, impurity of the blood, kidney disease, asthma, bronchitis, etc. At certain times he drives through the streets in a cart drawn by four horses. It is no surprise that a number of the curious are drawn to this event. Yesterday night the Miracle Doctor (as he is called by the common people around here) began his activities, which consists of massaging rheumatic sufferers. Only one patient showed up. The "miracle doctor" plans to stay here for about three weeks. Healing is free of charge. Everyone who seeks a cure for rheumatism has only to come to him to obtain complete healing. Only when the results of his treatment have been witnessed will he sell his remedies, such as Sequah-oil which costs one guilder a bottle, as well as the Indian prairie flower and another remedy that will immediately heal all internal pains. He will help the poor and they will obtain a free bottle, even two when necessary. To avoid deception he asks for a note from a minister of the Church, confirming that the person is really poor.[12]

Davenport soon featured in the national press as well. A week after the local newspaper report the *Nieuwe Rotterdamsche Courant* wrote:

> Every night the miracle doctor is driven to the market place in his golden cart, drawn by four beautiful horses and accompanied by music. The sick who are even brought to him in bed are treated on the spot by rubbing them with

> Sequah oil. At night the community is understandingly very excited to see him. Naturally he performs miracle cures.[13]

Davenport's cart was indeed a gaudy affair, akin to a circus wagon. It was adorned all over with statues of Red Indians, paintings and mirrors. It was designed in red and lavishly finished in gold. In it a six-men-strong brass band was seated, dressed up in Indian gear. The healer himself wore a Mexican-style leather outfit and a broad-rimmed cowboy hat.

The medical inspector of the district of Zeeland and the west of Noord-Brabant, where Roozendaal was located, could hardly fail to take notice of Davenport's activities. In a letter to the Minister of the Interior he asked whether Sequah should not be expelled from the country. The Minister replied, however, that this was not in accordance with the immigration law. The inspector had to be satisfied that, in order to indict Davenport in the magistrates' court of Bergen-op-Zoom, he could be charged with the illegal practice of medicine and the unlicensed sale of medicines. When the case was tried at the end of August, the healer had already departed for Rotterdam. In any case, convictions do not seem to have worried him unduly, since on appeal he was fined only one hundred and fifty guilders.[14] Nonetheless, as a response to such policing he hired shortly afterwards a licensed doctor to cover the medical side of his dealings. He procured also the services of a registered pharmacist to sell his oil. Davenport's sales route was cleverly chosen. Roozendaal may have been a minor town but it occupied a strategic position at the intersection of the route from Flushing (in the 1890s the port of arrival for ships from England) into the interior, with the route from Antwerp northwards to Rotterdam. The healer's itinerary carried him directly into the main towns of the Netherlands without venturing into the 'backward' countryside, rightly expecting the sufferers to flock to the market towns. After performing his healing in Rotterdam, he travelled straight to Amsterdam, in direct challenge to the Dutch medical profession.

## The Treatment

IN ROTTERDAM DAVENPORT MANAGED eventually to attract considerable attention, although only after several attempts. Already the first performance drew a 'large public of diverse rank and file' attracted no doubt by leaflets distributed from the advertising wagon and the sensational performance. A patient apparently unable to walk was carried onto the stage. As one of the Rotterdam papers described the event: 'Sequah immediately took away the man's cane and broke it in pieces, saying that he wouldn't need it anymore'. Behind a curtain the man was undressed, massaged and put on his feet again. A journalist, who had been admitted into the secluded area, described the patient:

> Now he had to make gymnastic movements, because he was still afraid of moving his feet. At first the man hardly dared to use his legs fearing the pains that cut through the bone and which had already plagued him for six weeks. But soon he moved more freely and with a bright face he began to dance and jump. He was told to jump still higher and landed on his feet ever more forcefully. For his blood to flow through his veins more quickly Sequah raised the man three feet high from the floor and then dropped him.

The patient put on his clothes and was then displayed to the public when he even attempted some dancing steps to the beat of the music. After that he was given some money. The next day, he was reported as having gone for an hour's walk, 'with much success, as he told us'.[15] The public quickly became aware that something very special was happening around Davenport. 'Even the competition from the fair does not harm him', the *Rotterdamsche Courant* remarked. Soon enterprising figures tried to join the bandwagon. Some started a business in salad oil, 'pretending it was Sequah-oil'. Others even went as far as stealing the real thing, Sequah oil, from the premises where Davenport held his performances. In Moerdijk, a small village south of Rotterdam, a Sequah impersonator gave an open-air show and there was even a plant named after him.[16]

Sequah, the healer, soon became a household name. Nevertheless, his fame was established on a particular day, 26 August 1891, from whence newspaper coverage of his performances increased dramatically. There were several reasons for this. A special Sequah issue of the *Monthly for the Repression of Quackery* was published on that day. It launched a fierce attack on Davenport, calling him 'a foreign quack, who exploits the suffering of miserable patients'. At the same time a ban was also issued on the sale of Davenport's bottles with remedies and the Rotterdam police started criminal proceedings against him.[17] The authorities conspired to put the spotlight on the healer. Yet it could not deflect from his public appeal, as it was expressed in December 1891, the next occasion on which there was an attempt to prosecute him:

> Sequah has confused every professor, doctor and pharmacist. At first the newspapers were taken to task by some doctors because they wrote about Sequah and thus gave him free publicity; the *Monthly for the Repression of Quackery* acquired some of the same medicine (...) Sequah acquired public favour! Sequah was celebrated, more than a *doctor*, more than a *professor*, even

more than a *monarch* – and this caused the jealousy of the *medical faculty*! But however they put up arms against Sequah, they could not rob him of the gratitude of the patients who were delivered from their suffering![18]

## The Healer's Impact

SEQUAH'S TOUR THROUGH THE NETHERLANDS only lasted a little over two years. It virtually ended in the summer of 1893 when a lingering conflict with the company came to a head. Subsequently, Davenport severed his links and started his own enterprise. In the autumn of the same year he settled in The Hague where he stayed until 1901 when he moved back to London. Thereafter he disappeared from historical scrutiny.

Everywhere Davenport went as Sequah he attracted enormous crowds, a lot of attention and much debate. This is witnessed by over eight hundred reports from many local Dutch newspapers about the events he staged and the reactions he provoked. One of his public's popular pastimes was to unharness the horses of his carriage and to pull it by hand through the streets, as in a triumphal procession. It was copied everywhere in the Netherlands. It was a routine not unique to the Netherlands for British Sequahs were similarly treated which suggests the company had a hand in its transmission.[19] In the end, Sequah left such a deep and lasting impression that, years later, he was still considered the ultimate 'quack' and the worst nightmare of every campaigner against quackery. The *Monthly for the Repression of Quackery* in 1908, for example, feared the rise of a 'new Sequah' as they called a healer with similar intentions to Davenport. Again, during the debates in 1914 concerning the abolition of the medical monopoly, Sequah figured among the few healers who were actually named by doctors as a warning example in their opposition to the campaign of Protestant lawyers to turn medicine into a free trade. As late as 1925, the Chief Inspector of Public Health remarked that no other healer had staged shows that resembled Sequah's performances.[20] Sequah also survived in the memory of his patients and he was celebrated in rhymes and songs.[21] A rhyme recorded in 1960 in Frisia, for example, almost seventy years after his grand tour suggests a long folk memory:

> Have you read in a certain newspaper
> That Zeekwa has arrived in our fatherland
> When you have crooked legs or are bothered by rheumatism
> Come along to Zeekwa who will cure you with music
> Are you bothered by lice or flees in your neck
> Come along to Zeekwa who will catch them with his cap.[22]

The last two lines are somewhat enigmatic. They are partly dictated by the rhyme and partly a joke but, at the same time, they refer to Sequah's 'carnivalesque' performance and to his association with the lower classes, signified by the cap. Another instance of how the healer was remembered was voiced in 1962. A farmer in the province of Limburg told an interviewer how he had heard many yarns about Sequah: 'Because he was not allowed to practise as a doctor himself, he used the services of his assistant, Dr Davenport. Once he performed in Venlo, at the Hotel National. Beforehand he held a musical procession through the town and handed sweets to all the children. He treated his patients with many words and with music'.[23] Apart from the confusion of names, which tells us that the doctor who accompanied Sequah was pure 'window-dressing', the memory of the farmer, though selective, was fairly accurate.

## Popularity Reviewed

HOW CAN SEQUAH'S ENORMOUS POPULARITY be explained, a popularity unsurpassed in the Netherlands for almost a century? Can his case throw light on the attraction of other 'irregular' or 'alternative' healers? Why did so many people flock to his shows after their initial hesitation? Why did Davenport sell thousands of bottles of his oil?[24]

There are no simple answers to these questions. The reasons for the appeal of 'alternative medicine' seem to be sufficiently complex that the Dutch governmental Committee on Alternative Treatments, which recently investigated the effectiveness of all kinds of non-regular cures, decided to refrain completely from asking these kinds of questions.[25] Popularity, however, is the most important factor in understanding the success of 'quackery'. Most cures of 'irregular healers', to put it differently, are ascribed nowadays to pure suggestion or the so-called placebo effect, as indeed was the case a century ago when this was a favourite argument used by the opponents of 'quackery'. Nevertheless, this does not preclude studying why 'alternative medicine' was so attractive to sufferers.[26] Precisely because the placebo effect is deemed to play a very important part in processes of healing a cultural approach becomes essential.[27] This calls for a shift in approach, from thinking in terms of verifiable numbers to considering changing attitudes and impressions by people of specific age, class, education and gender and to specific situations.

In the course of this research on irregular healers, it has become clear that it makes little sense to identify general conditions of the rise and fall of a healer's popularity. Different healers seem to have pursued different strategies. Analysis of individual healers even reveals different aspects of popularity. The case of Peter Stegeman, also known as 'the peasant from Staphorst', provides one example.[28] The way this healer communicated with his patients appears to have been of vital importance for his appeal. He always gave them a great deal of attention, expressed himself in simple language and kept his physical distance; he never touched his patients but only looked at them with his piercing eyes. Furthermore, he only asked to be paid for his remedies not for his advice which he gave freely. The 'renegade' doctor, as anti-quacks referred to such a 'collaborator', who shielded him from persecution for a couple of years, in contrast, did touch the patients and spoke in Latin which his patients perceived as incomprehensible sounds.[29] Yet, Stegeman's specific pattern of direct communication between healer and patient does not seem to have been applicable to another very famous early twentieth-century Dutch healer, the urologist Pieter van Bijsterveldt, who attained proverbial status in and around Rotterdam.[30] He subscribed also to the inalienability and integrity of the individual body but, instead of looking at his patients and talking to them, he treated them from a distance.[31] His method of 'piss-gazing' made this possible and did not require his physical presence. Whatever the differences in communication and diagnosis, both Van Bijsterveldt and Stegeman were orthodox Protestants, as probably was a substantial portion of their patients.

A healer's popularity was linked usually to his or her use of speech within the specific setting of the medical encounter. This is not only apparent if it is considered that a regular doctor's medical prestige derived at least partly from his professional clothing, his use of Latin and his illegible handwriting. It is also clear from the practices of somnambules. These women healers derived their popularity amongst others from their oracular speech, uttered in a trance. This was complete gobbledegook for their intellectual opponents, but for their patients it struck the right balance between authority and understanding.[32] Indeed, what is to be made of Davenport, an Englishman, who at least at the start of his stay in the Netherlands did not speak the Dutch language and who needed an interpreter whenever he addressed his audience? How could he possibly have communicated with his audience and have persuaded them of his healing power and that of his remedy?

## The Language of Quackery

SEQUAH, THE MOST FAMOUS and flamboyant healer in the Netherlands, derived his reputation from the way he communicated with his potential customers, using visual and audio aids. People did not see a cart like his every day and they were intrigued also to witness a massage on stage as a form of entertainment, especially if the majority of the public was barred by a curtain from seeing exactly what happened on stage, thereby rendering the scene more mysterious. While this was happening Sequah's musical band entertained the public. Evil tongues whispered that the sound of music served to stifle the screams of the sufferers when they were rubbed rather roughly with the oil. When he was confronted with this criticism the healer immediately gave a performance without any music. However, he found it necessary to hide naked parts of the patient's body from the general public, although journalists and doctors were invited to step behind the curtain; the healing process after all needed impartial witnesses who would be able to tell the world about it. What was very visible to the public, nevertheless, were people who had been formerly tormented by rheumatism and who were now miraculously healed after their treatment by Sequah. They were seen throwing away their sticks and crutches and even dancing on stage. Davenport went as far as organising occasional running contests between those he had successfully cured. This was to prove that his cure lasted beyond one theatrical evening. Davenport was also an inspired speaker. Such were his oratorical skills that he was urged to run for parliament, not only in the Netherlands but also in Scotland where he had been active in 1890.[33] According to one of the Liberal newspapers, 'Sequah even outshines Domela Nieuwenhuis'.[34] Although Davenport needed an interpreter on stage, this man merely provided subtitles to the healer's compelling performance. Yet, being an acclaimed orator who was able to counter the attacks of his opponents with wit did not necessarily make him a sympathetic communication partner who inspired confidence. Nevertheless, he shared with other irregular healers the ability and the habit to speak the language people understood. All popular healers revered their patients' own views and feelings. This is where they laid the burden of diagnosis. 'They tell me they are in pain', Davenport said, 'and I believe them. Ladies and gentlemen, when you are suffering from headache and the doctor comes to visit you, how is he to know what you are suffering from unless you tell him?' It was Davenport's supreme achievement, in the medical encounter on stage, that he bridged opposites: between healer and public, between the stage and the floor, between the fully dressed and the naked, between illness and cure. Thus, he was able to convey a sense of wholeness and harmony.[35]

## The Image of Christ

BEYOND THE ANALYSIS of the direct communication between healer and patient it is also possible to indicate a deeper cultural reason for Davenport's popularity. His actions were, in fact, easily associated with the image of Christ the healer. This was for a number of reasons. One being that Davenport applied the method of laying on of hands rather like Jesus Christ and described in the gospel of Mark, 6:5. 'What you did to me is a miracle', a woman from Venlo told him and many would have agreed with her.[36] This comparison with Jesus Christ may sound far-fetched but less so if it is considered that, in different contexts, it has been made in relation to other healers.[37] Moreover, there are sufficient grounds for the conclusion that many of Sequah's followers subscribed openly to this notion and that others recognised it implicitly. Indeed, it is quite likely that the healer himself deliberately engineered it.

The extract from a national newspaper quoted at the beginning of this paper contains a clue to this sentiment: the sick were brought to 'Sequah' in a bed, it was written, which evokes the image of Lazarus brought to Jesus (Mark 2:3–4). A satirical piece from the weekly paper *De Amsterdammer* makes the biblical connection even clearer. This starts with the words: 'And in those days it came to pass...'. A few more passages underline the biblical style:

> Then came a man from a foreign country sitting in a wagon of gold, with music and resoundings, and the fame of his deeds proceeded him, for he had healed many and he had made walk those who had sat down in sadness. (...) Then the old and the young fell on their knees and called the name of Sequah in ecstasy and started to praise him with hymns and prayers'.[38]

In this context it is of little concern that the author of this article probably wanted to ridicule the healer and his adherents; what is of significance is the way it was done. Others used even more direct messianic connotations, like a minister in the Calvinist town of Dordrecht. He said, during one of Sequah's performances: 'God has taken him to be a staff in his hand to cure the suffering mankind'. Sequah, he declared, was an 'envoy of God' and, in the following months, this phrase was repeated regularly in the publications of the Society for the Repression of Quackery. Sequah's divine gift was still remembered many years later.[39] 'What do you think about this deification of Sequah?' wrote a critic to one of the newspapers from Noord-Brabant. The same man also thought that people visited Sequah's performances 'to admire the only and immortal hero in his halo of supremacy and bliss'.[40]

Davenport shrewdly exploited the rumours of his supernatural gifts to his advantage: he appeared modest by denying them explicitly while at the same time he reinforced them through carefully staged symbolic actions. Thus, he was reported to have said in Dordrecht: 'I am not God's envoy – as a certain minister told you this week; I am only an ordinary human being who asks you to believe what I am saying'.[41] This did not stop him from introducing a new element in his show in the very town in which he was denying his divinity. He not only healed the lame and the crippled but also started to feed the poor and to quench the thirsty in Dordrecht. Men, women and children in need, each in turn, were offered, from then on, a free meal in every town he visited. At the same time they were also given special gifts, usually donated by the local shopkeepers. The public responded, during the evenings, with flowers, poems and all kinds of presents for Sequah. The reporter of the *Algemeen Handelsblad*, another national newspaper, described the scene in Dordrecht:

> On Monday night he was presented with a big wreath, made of yellow roses and laurel leafs. On the ribbons was printed in Dutch and in English: "When you arrived in the Netherlands, it was proclaimed: Do not believe him. He may kill you. Many inhabitants from Dordrecht now call out to you: O God, protect the saviour of the rheumatic sufferers and the benefactor of the poor!" When this wreath was laid upon Sequah's shoulders a huge cheer erupted. "Long shall he live in glory"! sounded from every mouth. (...)
>
> On Tuesday night Sequah received a neat bouquet of white lilacs. In the name of some prominent citizens, who wished to remain anonymous, he was also presented with a poem, which went as follows:
>> To raise the spirit of the suppressed,
>> To comfort those who grieve,
>> To help those who weep,
>> To quench those who are hungry,
>> To bless with your best gifts,
>> Is a duty but also bliss![42]

The perception of Sequah's performance conformed to the contemporary image of Jesus Christ. This made Sequah appear like the Messiah sent by God to evict the usurers, the official doctors, from the temple of healing. Like Jesus he was perceived also as a martyr and the attacks from the Society for the Repression of Quackery and from legal authorities only strengthened this image. Sequah was said to act as a 'benefactor of mankind, a noble friend of humanity' and all those who took the trouble to attend his shows, which many did, could see with their own eyes how he healed the sick and invited the children to come to him (Mark 10:14).

Finally, the circumstances in which Davenport operated, just before the turn of the century, contributed to his impact; given the importance of liminal time in Christian ideology. This was noticed also by contemporaries:

> Those, who have lived through this craze already for some time as well as those who have never experienced it may find it hard to imagine that the "fin de siècle" city of The Hague runs to the Sequah-agent, as if he were a miraculous human being, rather like Paris celebrated Mesmer a good hundred years ago.[43]

## Resolution

DAVENPORT'S EXPERIENCE WITH THE LAW was very symptomatic of that of other famous healers. Once he had managed to exploit the loopholes in the legal system he was essentially left untroubled. He visited about thirty towns, during his two year's tour, but he was prosecuted only in the first three. The third case in Amsterdam depended upon the doctor who covered him having left the stage for a few minutes. Davenport paid the fines very readily. About nine months after his stay in Amsterdam he was once again prosecuted in Groningen, this time merely because his arrival at that town coincided with the conviction of a local masseur. The Groningen court eventually acquitted Davenport on appeal.[44] Davenport, for his part, hit back at his main public opponents. He sued the Society for the Repression of Quackery for libel, even though this organisation was only indirectly responsible for the prosecutions against him. He also won this case. When the most notorious 'quack' was able to practice almost unhindered, it can be safely assumed that healers of lesser renown could fare even better. If they were popular enough to be prosecuted, they also earned enough money to pay the fines or they had supporters who paid the fines for them. Laws which were meant to curtail the illegal practice of medicine turned out to promote healers by giving them free publicity, rather than by putting a stop to their trade. In the Netherlands, a country that was envied by medical associations abroad for possessing stringent medical laws, fighting 'quackery' often amounted to fighting metaphorical windmills. Of course, fighting God's envoy was sheer sacrilege.

*An earlier version of this paper has been published in Dutch under the title: 'De Godsgezant. Over de populariteit van een irreguliere genezer', Groniek. Historisch tijdschrift 131 (1995), 198–208. I would like to thank the Wellcome Trust for providing me with the means to consult the British sources. Cornelie Usborne's help in reformulating the original text was invaluable.*

# Notes

1 Roy Porter, *The Greatest Benefit to Mankind. A Medical History of Humanity from Antiquity to the Present* (London, 1997), p. 284; Matthew Ramsey, 'The Politics of Professional Monopoly in Nineteenth-Century Medicine: The French Model and Its Rivals' in Gerald L. Geison (ed.), *Professions and the French State* (Philadelphia, 1984), 225–305.

2 It could be argued that since the British Medical Act of 1858 did not outlaw medicine by non-licensed practitioners and because of the proliferation of social history of medicine in Britain, there is little incentive to study the prosecution of illegal practitioners. A mere glance at the *British Medical Journal*, however, suggests this to be wrong. It reveals the many different pretexts under which 'quacks', in fact, could be prosecuted also in Britain.

3 *Maandblad tegen de Kwakzalverij* 34 (1914) nr. 1, supplement.

4 Roy Porter, 'Quacks. An unconscionable time dying' in Susan Budd & Ursula Sharma (eds.), *The Healing Bond. The patient-practitioner relationship and therapeutic responsibility* (London & New York, 1994), pp. 63–81, quote 65.

5 Cf. Jens Lachmund & Gunnar Stolberg, *Patientenwelten. Krankheit und Medizin vom späten 18. bis zum frühen 20. Jahrhundert im Spiegel von Autobiographien* (Opladen, 1995).

6 Cf. Marijke Gijswijt-Hofstra, 'Homeopathy's early Dutch conquests: the Rotterdam Clientele of Clemens von Bönninghausen in the 1840s and 1850s', *Journal of the History of Medicine and Allied Sciences* 51 (1996), 155–83.

7 For some regions of Europe legend texts contain valuable information, cf. Willem de Blécourt, 'Duivelbanners in de noordelijke Friese Wouden, 1860–1930', *Volkskundig bulletin* 14 (1988), 159–87. See also Torunn Selberg, 'Personal narratives on healing', *Fabula* 31 (1990), 284–8.

8 To distinguish him from his colleagues elsewhere, I have called him 'the Dutch Sequah'.

9 H.J.W. Drooglever Fortuyn, *Kwakzalverij, bijgeloof en geneeskunst* (Amsterdam, 1940), p. 42.

10 *The Chemist and Druggist*, 22 August 1891, 318.

11 Wellcome Institute for the History of Medicine, Sequah archives, box 1, file 2/G, Norman to Kasper, 18 June 1891.

12 *De Grondwet*, 18 July 1891.

13 *Nieuwe Rotterdamsche Courant*, 25 June 1891.

14 ARA (The Hague), Archive 'medische politie', inv.nr. 20, nrs. 2373, 2465, 2490; *Mededeelingen omtrent het Geneeskundig Staatstoezicht in de inspectie Zeeland en westelijk Noord-Brabant*, meeting 15 December 1891, pp. 17, 21; *Weekblad van het Recht* 6087; Rijksarchief Noord-Brabant ('s-Hertogenbosch), Archive 'arrondissementsrechtbank Breda', inv.nr. 205, nr. 626.

15  Citations are taken from the *Maasbode* and the *Rotterdamsch Nieuwsblad* of 29 July 1891. See also *De Tijd* of the same date.

16  *Rotterdamsche Courant*, 14 August; *Nieuwe Rotterdamsche Courant*, 4 August; *Rotterdamsch Nieuwsblad*, 6 August; *NRC*, 14 and 15 August; *Rotterdamsche Courant*, 16/17 August; *de Maasbode*, 21 August; *NRC*, 2 September 1891.

17  *Rotterdamsch Nieuwsblad*, 26, 28 August; *Rotterdamsche Courant*, 28, 30/31 August; *NRC*, 28, 29, 30 August 1891.

18  *Asmodée*, 31 December 1891.

19  Cf. W. Schupbach, 'Sequah; an English "American medicine"-man in 1890', *Medical history* 29 (1985), 272–317, esp. 296.

20  *Maandblad tegen de kwakzalverij*, 28 (1908) nrs. 3 and 4, 32 (1912) nr. 3; 45 (1925) nr. 4; *Nederlandsch tijdschrift voor geneeskunde*, 30 May 1914, p. 2023, 2028.

21  In 1891 there were even plays written about him but it is not known to this author whether they were also performed.

22  Archive Meertens-Institute (Amsterdam), ms. Joh. Boonstra. The rhyme is given here in translation.

23  Archive Meertens-Institute, collection Engels, nr. 50. Cf. *Dagblad voor Noord-Limburg*, 29 December 1961; Henk Kooijman, *Volksverhalen uit het grensgebied van Zuid-Holland, Utrecht, Gelderland en Noord-Brabant* (Amsterdam, 1988), nr. 1111; *Volkskunde-atlas voor Nederland en Vlaams-België*, *Commentaar*, II (Antwerp, 1965), 78–9.

24  Exact sales figures are not available. According to the Society for the Repression of Quackery, at the end of October 1891 40,000 crates with 300 or 400 bottles each had already been imported.

25  See the report of the 'Gezondheidsraad' (Health Council), *Alternatieve behandelwijzen en wetenschappelijk onderzoek* (Den Haag 1993).

26  Cf. Cecil G. Hellman, *Culture, health and illness* (Oxford, 1994), pp. 196–201.

27  Cf. Paul Unschuld, 'The Conceptual Determination (Überformung) of Individual and Collective Experiences of Illness' in Caroline Currer & Margaret Stacey (eds.), *Concepts of Health, Illness and Disease. A Comparative Perspective* (Providence and Oxford, 1986).

28  In this context 'peasant' (Dutch: *boertje*) had come to signify: 'healer from the countryside'.

29  Willem de Blécourt, 'Het Staphorster boertje. De geneeskundige praktijk van Peter Stegeman (1840–1922)' in Marijke Gijswijt-Hofstra (ed.), *Geloven in genezen* (Amsterdam, 1991), 171–94.

30  Ewoud Sanders & Rob Tempelaars, *Krijg de vinkentering! 1001 Nederlandse en Vlaamse verwensingen* (Amsterdam/Antwerp, 1998), pp. 116–7.

31 Willem de Blécourt, 'The Tale of Two Brothers. Urine diagnosis and medical politics in the Netherlands and Michigan, early twentieth century', paper given at the SSHM conference, *Medicine and the Family*, University of Exeter, 1995.

32 Willem de Blécourt, *Het Amazonenleger. Irreguliere genezeressen in Nederland, 1850–1930* (Amsterdam, 1999), chapter 6.

33 *The Greenock Herald*, 5 April 1890, cf. *Nieuwe Bredasche Courant*, 29 March 1893.

34 Ferdinand Domela Nieuwenhuis was the contemporary Dutch epitome of the public orator; a former Protestant minister turned socialist and later anarchist.

35 Willem de Blécourt, 'Sequah in Amsterdam. Over de invloed van reclame op een medische markt', *Focaal. Tijdschrift voor antropologie* 21 (1993), 131–72.

36 *Limburger Koerier*, 13 January 1893.

37 Cf. Selberg, 'Personal narratives', 286; Herbert Schäfer, *Der Okkulttäter* (Hamburg 1959), 140.

38 *De Amsterdammer*, 11 October 1891.

39 *Dordrechts Nieuwsblad*, 28 January 1892; *Maandblad tegen de kwakzalverij*, 12 (1892) nrs. 3 and 4; 13 (1893) nr. 9; J. van Riel, 'Geschiedkundig overzicht der Vereeniging over de jaren 1880–1905' in *Gedenkboek van de Vereeniging tegen de kwakzalverij* (Dordrecht 1906), 160–97, esp. 177.

40 *Noord Brabanter*, 11 November 1892.

41 *Nieuwe Rotterdamsche Courant*, 30 January 1892.

42 *Algemeen Handelsblad*, 5 February 1892. See also *NRC*, 2 and 3 February 1892.

43 *Nieuws van den Dag*, 29 February 1892.

44 Willem de Blécourt, 'Irreguliere genezers in de stad Groningen in de tweede helft van de 19e eeuw', *Gronings Historisch jaarboek* 1 (1994), 126–41.

# Female Voices in Male Courtrooms – Abortion Trials in Weimar Germany

## Cornelie Usborne

THE PRACTICE AND PROSECUTION of abortion in the early twentieth century is a central concern both for the social historian of medicine and the social historian of crime. For the former because, as a social practice, abortion touches on an essential part of women's health – reproductive choice and the problems associated with this choice – and because it was here that the medical profession fought hard to assert its influence for policy making and to gain a monopoly in regulating and treating it. For the social historian of crime abortion constitutes a challenging problem. It was, next to infanticide, which it replaced in importance in the twentieth century, the most gender-specific crime. In addition, it was one which attracted the most controversy as one of the key delicts to efforts at criminal law reform in the early twentieth century, and what was thought of its exceptionally low detection rate, largely because of the gap between official retribution and popular tolerance. Of course, men also often had a big part in abortion, both as instigators and procurers, and they were questioned by the police and in court as witnesses or charged and punished as accomplices. But women were always far more central in the event and, in the 1920s and 1930s, both as aborting women and as abortionists, particularly as lay abortionists.

Weimar Germany (1918–1933) was not exceptional in its legal attitudes towards abortion,[1] but it was exceptional in the number of women estimated to have undergone abortions – in 1930 the number of abortions was estimated at one million, thereby being higher than the number of births. In addition, although abortion was a subject of concern in all

European countries during the early twentieth century, in no other place did it attract such passionate public attention and capture the attention of politicians, feminists, sex reformers, novelists, dramatists and poets. Germany displayed more clearly than any other western European country the tension between an authoritarian law rooted in a traditional conception of women's role and a society in rapid transformation in which women's modern lifestyle undermined such attitudes. The rapid decline in the secular birth rate and the growing annual rate of estimated abortions propelled the question of fertility control into the public limelight. The vociferous campaign for abortion law reform and the quest by doctors to medicalise abortion ensured that the topic remained one of the most contested issues of public health, of women's rights and of party politics.[2] Yet, public perceptions and private experience were rarely the same. Even the most ardent reformer usually considered an abortion to be an unfortunate social necessity, albeit one to be overcome with welfare and better access to contraception rather than by the heavy-handed threats of the law. Nevertheless, for many thousands of women of childbearing age, the termination of an unwanted pregnancy was, in the 1920s and early 1930s, an everyday experience which they had either undergone themselves or of which they had intimate knowledge through neighbours, friends and family members. Despite the attention which the issue of abortion has received in the liberal era of the Weimar Republic,[3] the social history of abortion, written with a view from below, remains to be documented.[4]

Most historians have concentrated on public policies and public discourse in which abortion usually features as either an unacceptable crime or a necessary evil. However, contrary to official views, most women did not necessarily regard it as a disaster. A termination of an unwanted pregnancy was not only a last resort for them but also a routine form of birth control. Abortion appealed because it was practical and cost-effective, especially when compared with the available contraceptives which needed forethought, regular application and often medical help. This made them, in the long run, costly and time consuming. Contraceptives, of course, were not always reliable. This notwithstanding, public discourse usually presented abortion as a tragedy. Despite the strides women's emancipation had made since the First World War, the dominant ideology in the 1920s remained that pregnancy and childbirth were women's destiny and that most women also desired to become mothers, albeit under the right circumstances. Thus, abortion was considered officially as a complete reversal of all that was positive about reproduction. The termination of a pregnancy was judged as murder by the Church. According to the penal code it was a crime (at least until 1926), by most state authorities it was regarded as a sign of immorality, and Germany's Medical Association viewed it with disdain.[5] It is true that women themselves often associated abortion with danger to their health, with fear of detection, with embarrassment in persuading an abortionist and with possible isolation from family and friends. Yet, measured against the even bigger problem of an unwanted pregnancy, abortion was also regarded by many women as a welcome release and the abortionist as a helpmate.

It is this dichotomy between the private views of aborting women and their accomplices, and the official line of the judiciary and other public commentators, that is at the centre of this paper, which is part of a larger project on cultures of abortion in Weimar and Nazi Germany and based, amongst other sources, on the close study of criminal abortion cases in various areas, Catholic and Protestant, agricultural and industrial, rural and urban. These sources will be used in conjunction with contemporary newspaper reports, doctors' case books, diaries and reminiscences. This paper concentrates on a particular case study which will be complemented by and supported with information gleaned from other judicial cases. The primary concern is to show how a criminal abortion case was constructed out of at least two competing discourses, on the one hand that of the aborting woman and her accomplices, and on the other that of the law enforcement agencies whose agenda was quite different. It is argued that the woman's voice was still discernible at the beginning of the criminal investigation but that it was increasingly muffled and, in the end, curtailed and obscured by official pronouncements. The question of the authenticity of defendants' voices is problematic since their views are always mediated through the language of the scribe and shaped by the set of questions posed. Nevertheless, given that every opinion is situated and all individuals can only be understood in relation to their circumstances and in relation to those persons they live in close contact with, to the education received and to the culture around them, the opinion of women accused of abortion can be more or less reconstructed by carefully peeling away the layers of official language and making visible the framework of questions and suggestions in which their stories were told. On a number of occasions, female defendants are allowed to speak directly to the reader. This occurred when they rejected the official version of their interrogation and demanded that the wording be changed.

Such court cases, if they are fairly complete, which many of them are in Germany during the Weimar Republic, always provide a valuable insight into the everyday life of women during the 1920s and early 1930s. The concern is with this access to the very intimate sphere and the hope of being able to shed light on women's attitudes and experiences within their families, with their sweethearts or husbands, or in isolation from their kin and friends, that is so rarely open to historians rather than with the politics of abortion or the process of medicalisation of abortion explored elsewhere.[6] But although it is women's own appraisal of their situation and their actions which are of most interest, the judicial files offer also a new insight into official thinking. For example, they reveal the seemingly straightforward question of what it was that was criminalised by law and what it was that was the subject of the accusation to have been in reality far more complex and subtle than would at first appear. An anonymous letter written in Berlin in June 1929 and addressed to the local police station offers a good illustration:

> In the interest of the general public something should be done quickly to stop the dealings of Frau Martha Spitzer[7] of Berlinerst. 156. She charges 2 Marks for fortune telling using cards (*Kartenlegen*) which she uses to exploit people's emotional state which is after all why they are driven to go to a fortune-teller in the first place and she promises women that she can help them with sympathy. For this kind of swindle Spitzer charges 30–80 Mks. To women who recognise this swindle too late and ask for their money back she is insolent enough to deny outright that she ever received any. Spitzer lures mostly wives whose husbands have deserted them and young girls to whom she returns their sweetheart or else she promises to get rid of him when those concerned want to get rid of their lover. On these occasions women have to hand over material, for example bits of underwear (*Wäschestücke*) from their menfolk. She says she needs this so that she can work better against them. Such a sacrifice, as she calls it, must no longer be touched by the owners of this underwear: a trick so that as much as possible is handed over to her. Those who cannot pay in one lump sum must pay in instalments and in order to get her money on time Frau Spitzer threatens women with misfortune who do not pay on time but those who pay are promised instant relief.

The letter then urges the police to search Frau Spitzer's flat as soon as possible because rich evidence would be uncovered. If there was a delay this evidence might be hidden away. The letter continues:

> ... another thing, if women threaten her with the police she declares that nobody can harm her. She has so many friends among the police whom she has helped to return their wives and she carries with her a little silk pouch with the figure of Lucifer and whatever all the other devils are called that is why nobody can harm her not even in the courts. She says she has often been in court for abortions and similar matters and no judge could get at her because of this protection. It is like this that this woman carries on with her foul work and the time has now finally come to prevent her from harming even more people. Who knows how many years the woman has been carrying on with such doings and how many people have already been harmed... My records will be confirmed by

the house search I still want to keep my name secret because Frau Spitzer attacks one in the middle of the street....[8]

This then was a denunciation of a well-known female healer to the police for fraud. The writer of the letter was revealed later as a certain Frau Winzer whom Frau Spitzer suspected herself because she had had a quarrel with her in the street. Indeed, Frau Winzer had then threatened to ensure that Frau Spitzer would end up in the *Zuchthaus* (penal servitude).

This letter is a valuable source affording rare insights into the everyday life of lower-class women hinting at their beliefs, aspirations and fears. It also reveals the custom of alternative medicine in a working-class community at a time when the majority of the population had been insured for free medical care under Weimar Germany's wide-ranging health insurance system. Weimar Germany, and the capital Berlin in particular, is usually portrayed as the byword for modernity[9] and by the end of the 1920s German working-class women were shown to lead a thoroughly rationalised lifestyle.[10] Yet, maybe surprisingly, such customs as fortune telling which might be placed more naturally in the period of pre-industrial rural society continued to be practised.[11] What is more, the practice of fortune telling with cards (*Kartenlegen*) and sympathetic magic, or magnetic sympathy, as the letter writer referred to it, was apparently popular in working-class districts and, judging from the tone of the letter, not considered in itself extraordinary or suspect.[12] This piece of evidence and similar examples suggest that it would be wrong to assume that research into twentieth-century legal documents concerning abortion and birth control would tend to be dry and prosaic without yielding such rich narratives as Natalie Zemon Davies' letters of remission in sixteenth-century France analysed in her *Fiction in the Archives*.[13] The letter quoted above and the various records of police and judicial interrogations which supplement it contain a wealth of revealing details which offer a keyhole view of women's private lives in the past otherwise largely denied to historians. The letter quoted is doubly rare, because it affords an uninterrupted personal view, i.e. a woman's voice unmediated since the letter was unprompted by official enquiries, even though it was addressed to the authorities. Thus, Frau Winzer's agenda was entirely different from that of the subsequent police action. Frau Winzer had no problems with Frau Spitzer's abortion practice and she referred to it only in passing. The police, however, appropriated the denunciation for their own purposes: ignoring the complaint of fraud, a comparatively minor charge, they concentrated instead on the incidental allusion to criminal abortions, a major charge which could carry a sentence of penal servitude. The letter had clearly been motivated by revenge. Revenge by a former client or friend was one of the two principal reasons why illegal abortions and abortionists came to the notice of the authorities when they had previously been shielded by the protective silence of their neighbourhood. The other main reason was when the operation had resulted in a serious injury and had necessitated emergency medical help or had caused the death of the aborting woman and had involved a coroner.

In order to understand the difference between the female working-class culture in which abortion was a fairly routine event and an official culture in which it was a criminal offence and a threat to public health and population strength, it is important to note that Frau Winzer had only complained about Frau Spitzer's fortune telling and sympathetic magic. She herself had most probably used these services and felt disgruntled because her lover or husband had not returned to her. Instead of turning to another more effective fortune teller she decided to ask the police for help to revenge her sense of betrayal. This demonstrates, in addition, that the police were not always considered as an expression of hostile state authority but could indeed be used by working-class people for their own ends. The police, however, had a different remit and used Frau Winzer's complaint for their own purpose, that is to suppress the practice of criminal abortion rather than to lend support to Frau Winzer's complaint of this fortune teller's apparently fraudulent claims. They decided to survey and eventually to search Frau Spitzer's flat to find incriminating evidence of her abortion activities. They were indeed successful for, behind Frau Spitzer's stove, they found hidden a number of notebooks containing the addresses of female abortion patients and the sums of money they had been asked to pay. There were also a number of women's photographs. The end result was that a successful wise-woman (*weise Frau*), as she was referred to in the neighbourhood, was charged, tried and convicted for having procured at least 20 criminal abortions on a commercial basis and for attempted abortion on nine other women. Frau Spitzer, a woman of 53 with four grown-up children, was kept in pre-trial detention for six months and then sentenced to a further 18 months' imprisonment, as well as to the loss of all civil rights for three years and to the payment of the costs of the trial. All attempts to plead extenuating circumstances or for clemency were rejected.[14] Frau Spitzer's prosecution also engendered a massive police hunt to trace, interrogate and finally to try 29 of her alleged abortion clients. Unlike some other European countries which treated the aborting woman only as a trial witness,[15] in Germany she was also tried as a defendant and usually received a prison sentence; although this was often suspended or commuted to a fine. This has the advantage, for the historian, that German abortion cases yield extraordinarily rich information on many women's private history: in this case, not just Frau Spitzer's testimony is available but also the testimonies of her 29 co-defendants about whom full statements of their interviews by the police, the pre-trial investigation (*Untersuchungsgericht*) and the cross-examinations conducted during the main trial are extant. There are also reports by social workers and medical experts but these may reveal more about the assumptions and prejudices of the authorities than of the defendants.

In order to distil a woman's true voice careful attention needs to be paid to the way the criminal case was constructed. The defendants' own words were naturally obscured by the bureaucratic language and concerns. In the arena of the police station or the court room defendants always appear on the losing end of an unequal power relationship. Female defendants faced an additional disadvantage. It was usual for women in the dock to be scrutinised and judged only by men who were likely to have little first-hand experience or sympathy with the dilemma of an unwanted pregnancy and the decision to terminate it. At this time the police, public prosecutors, judges and medical experts were always male and even among jurors women were rare. Typically, at the criminal proceedings of the *Landgericht* III (regional superior court) in Berlin in 1930 Frau Spitzer and her patients faced altogether ten men: three male judges, a public prosecutor, a trainee lawyer (*Referendar*) and five male jurors. The sixth juror was a woman. Judgements were based on a law of 1871 which expressed the ideology of a patriarchal society according to which women's role was largely confined to the home without any substantial influence on lawmaking or law enforcement. In the 1920s the abortion law was widely believed to be out of date, but the judiciary in the Weimar Republic was well known for its right-wing and conservative attitudes. This and the dominance of males in the law enforcement process served to inhibit women defendants. Yet there were other reasons why they might have been intimidated to speak their mind freely, for the aborting woman (and even more so, the abortionist) on trial faced potential prison sentences and social disgrace. More importantly, there was a serious risk of prejudice to the aborting woman's dignity and privacy because her sex life and personal history were generally cruelly exposed by the public prosecutor determined to undermine her credibility before the jury. She faced the humiliation of being cross-examined about the most minute details of her abortion. In addition, reports by social workers of visits to the defendant's home were used to establish evidence of 'good' or 'bad' social and sexual behaviour. It is quite justified to suggest that often it was not so much the deed of abortion that women were accused of but, in general, of leading a loose and antisocial life by middle-class standards. A termination of pregnancy by a woman who was regarded otherwise as respectable was treated invariably with more leniency than by a woman whose domestic circumstances had met with opprobrium. It was the added pressure of the close scrutiny of the entire personal life which was to prove intolerable to many women. In the trial of Frau Spitzer and her patients, Anna Koch is a good example of a defendant for whom the embarrassing criminal investigations probably proved too much. She had only arrived recently in Berlin from Breslau and had taken a manual job. She was 26 and single when she found herself pregnant by a married man. When questioned by the police Anna admitted her termination straight away. The police, however, were not satisfied and pressed her into the following confession: 'Last year I had sexual intercourse with a gentlemen whose name and address I cannot name any more. Since my period was not as strong as normal I presumed I was pregnant ... I could not marry the man who had made me pregnant ...' Possibly as a response to a policeman's promptings, an attempt to find exonerating circumstances (in this case, genetic fears) for her deed she added: 'Only after I had become involved with him I knew that he was a strong drinker. Otherwise I would have carried the child.'[16] Anna was then asked to describe, in detail, the three attempts by Frau Spitzer to procure her abortion as well as the precise sensations felt during them. Without waiting for the trial proper Anna committed suicide by gassing herself in custody.

Even if the public was excluded from the main proceedings of many abortion trials the extent of such semipublic humiliation can only be understood if it is appreciated that the defendant stood before her male inquisitors as a young woman (Frau Spitzer's clients were either in their twenties or early thirties) and one known to have been sexually active and whose sexuality was associated with deviance either because of the abortion or because of an illicit liaison whose details were always required to be told. Women's stories and women's voices were likely, of course, to have been influenced by this confrontation in court. Yet women's thoughts were often also distorted because they were rephrased in official legal language by the scribes in police stations or courts, and they were naturally shaped also by the specific questions asked by their male interrogators who were guided by quite different concerns from those of the defendants. Whereas many women were keen to show that their deed had been both rational and practical or indeed the only option within specific circumstances, interrogators were concerned with effective policing and prosecution and the correct adjudication of blame. They wanted to find out who had decided on the abortion in the first place and who knew about it, or who helped with it, in order to prosecute all those guilty of inciting, aiding and abetting; all punishable under German law. Or there were enquiries about precise financial transactions made between the aborting woman and her abortionist since abortion on a commercial basis carried extra-heavy penalties.[17] At a time before reliable pregnancy tests existed, women suspects were pressed to comment on the details of the aborted matter to prove, beyond doubt, that they had been pregnant in the first place and had undergone a termination rather than attempted to bring on a late period (even though an attempted abortion was, in theory at least, also a punishable offence). Frau Spitzer, for example, was asked repeatedly about the payment she had received. Referring to her account books with her patients' names, addresses and the sums of money she had demanded for the operation she said: 'I protest having carried out abortions for money. The money was given to me voluntarily. If one suggests that according to my book the sum was always 85 RM (a large sum for working-class women) and that the uniformity of the sum indicates that I have always demanded 85 RM let me point out that the addresses were written by the women themselves and that they saw therefore that other women before them had paid this sum. I only asked them to note down their addresses so that I could check how they were doing after the operation.'[18] Frau Spitzer did indeed visit her patients to see whether they had recovered from their miscarriages and whether the afterbirth had been expelled. This and the next statement (reduced in the judicial record to just one short sentence) were much more her own, and of course that of the women clients, rather than the interviewers' concern. After all, Frau Spitzer's reputation and her ability to make money from her abortion practice rested on her record of medical success. Frau Spitzer declared: 'I have never heard that a single person has died as a consequence of the operation.'[19] This is a rather understated reference to her considerable achievement that the many abortions she had induced had never caused any injury, let alone death, and that her female patients expressed their satisfaction frequently adding that they experienced no discomfiture. Frau Spitzer's record, thus, was admirable despite the fact that she had not studied medicine nor midwifery. She was entirely self-taught, having learnt about anatomy and abortion from the manuals of her mother, a trained midwife. It was a particularly proud achievement in the context of the public debate at the time which was dominated by the medical profession. Doctors usually blamed the consistently high levels of maternal mortality on criminal, especially lay, abortion.[20] Yet, of course, there were also important legal implications for Frau Spitzer's record, for abortion which ended in death was punishable with a minimum of 10 years' imprisonment.

Despite the many factors inhibiting women from giving their own
account much can be learnt from their unwitting testimony. For example,
Frau Margarete Schmalzer, another of Frau Spitzer's patients, revealed how
abortion was often planned long before the need arose. Schmalzer, a married
woman, worked as a white-collar employee in the electrical industry. At the
time she found herself pregnant she was only 24 but already had a three-year-
old child. She and her husband had not yet managed to rent their own flat
and the family relied on her salary. Thus, she was not yet ready to have a
second child. She explained how she came across Frau Spitzer's name as an
abortionist: 'I became aware of Frau Spitzer through Frau Schmidt (who
lived just round the corner). I spoke to Frau Schmidt and in the course of a
conversation she mentioned that Frau Spitzer also did abortions. At that
time I was not yet pregnant.'[21] Here, not only the existence of a female
network of self-help but also the long-term planning for family limitation are
discovered. Other examples are available of such a preventive strategy,
confirming that many working-class women shared the kind of rationalised
behaviour, i.e. taking control of their body and their personal fate, that is
commonly associated with the more middle-class New Woman of the
Weimar Republic. Asked by a criminal police officer to describe the abortion
process itself Margarete Schmalzer displayed a surprising knowledge of
medical and anatomical facts. When questioned about the results of her
miscarriage she said: 'The foetus was roughly 10 cm long. Spitzer had told me
to return with it so that she could see whether everything had gone
(*abgegangen*). But I did not find her at home and so I threw the foetus into
the loo.'[22] Such information indicates that Schmalzer's pregnancy was
advanced, probably five months, and that Frau Spitzer was surprisingly
prepared to induce a miscarriage at this late stage despite the greater risks
this involved. It also explains why she needed three attempts for the
intervention to succeed. But the statement also shows how pragmatic and
unsentimental ordinary women could be in dealing with their own foetus.
Their attitude is reminiscent of the women in the Bavarian countryside who
had committed infanticide at the turn of the century and who were studied
by Regina Schulte.[23] Schmalzer thought nothing of carrying an aborted
foetus through the streets of Berlin and then back home again, and
eventually dispensing with it as if it was normal bodily waste. Similarly, a
nineteen-year-old domestic servant, another of Frau Spitzer's patients,
thought it quite natural to ask a friend to run this errand for her. She and her
friend had originally gone together to Frau Spitzer to have their pregnancies
terminated. In fact, each helped with the other's operation. But in the case
of the friend the miscarriage had not occurred yet and since she needed to

return to Frau Spitzer for a second attempt, she did not appear to mind taking along her friend's parcel (the aborted foetus).[24]

Many of the abortion trials studied illustrate how the authorities attempted to re-reinforce existing gender stereotypes, such as the belief that women's testimony is less valid because they always react too emotionally to events while men always reaction rationally; or that women were caring and passive while men were assertive and active, etc. For example, a judge in a case of 1924 based his unexpected verdict entirely on his assumption of inborn gender characteristics.[25] The case concerned the former director of a gynaecological hospital in the Rhineland, a Dr Bauer, who was accused of illegal commercial abortions in seven cases, two of which had ended in death. The three medical experts could not agree as to whether the gynaecologist had performed the abortions in question legally or illegally, nor whether he was responsible for two fatalities which had resulted from his operations. One of the medical experts, Prof. Bumm from Berlin, the doyen of Germany's gynaecologists, relied more or less on Dr Bauer's own assertions; another expert was paid privately by Dr Bauer and unsurprisingly came to his defence. But the third medical expert, the director of another women's hospital in the Rhineland, made an impassioned plea on behalf of the two women who had died and accused the defendant of medical misconduct and gross negligence as, for example, he had failed to disinfect properly. He suggested also that the severe internal injuries which the autopsies had revealed were caused almost certainly by Dr Bauer's 'impatient' surgery.[26] Furthermore, Dr Bauer was found to have been given a previous warning by the local medical council which had long suspected him of illegal abortions.[27] The most damaging evidence, however, was the testimony of five women patients who confessed to having had abortions procured by Dr Bauer for money and who made clear that Dr Bauer was well known in the area 'to do it for money.'[28] Astonishingly Dr Bauer was acquitted of all charges. The judge justified his verdict with reference to the five women witnesses who were dismissed by him as unreliable because, as he put it, of women's natural tendency to confuse fact and fantasy. In the judge's own words: 'the defendant Dr Bauer does not seem very credible and despite Dr Bauer's solemn protestation of his own innocence the court is utterly convinced that he was indeed capable of having committed the criminal offences he is accused of; even though almost all the evidence speaks against him and although his co-defendants (i.e. his patients) and another female witness appeared infinitely more credible than Dr Bauer – nevertheless one cannot totally ignore that persons who have became pregnant illegitimately are especially prone to imagine events and subsequently believe strongly that they are true and then testify with genuine conviction objective non-truths as if they have actually taken place. This consideration alone persuaded the court to rule that Dr Bauer is not proven guilty beyond all doubt. He is thus acquitted on the grounds of insufficient evidence.'[29]

Research, on the other hand, shows that many female defendants undermined such gender stereotyping: they appeared not passive, but active, not docile but fiercely determined. There are quite a few incidents of women, young women among them, putting across strong views even under cross examination. Female defendants protested vigorously about incorrect statements produced by the scribe and demanded the wording be changed. Women also protested their innocence outspokenly and angrily. One defendant in the Spitzer case, for example, was only 25 and as a white-collar worker probably not highly educated, yet she was so outraged at having been wrongly implicated in the abortion scandal that she demanded compensation for slander.[30] Finally, abortion files reveal considerable emotional and practical co-operation between the sexes. Although abortion is usually considered as a woman's crime *par excellence* the experience of the operation and its punishment were rarely confined to women alone. Not only mothers, sisters or girlfriends but husbands, boyfriends, brothers, even fathers were much in evidence at the time leading up to, during and after the abortion. Under German law this made them accomplices and open to prosecution and punishment. In a famous case of 1924 a carpenter and his wife in Prussian Hesse stood accused of well over 60 criminal abortions in their own and the neighbouring villages. The case also involved 64 women defendants accused of having undergone abortions and 36 men accused of having helped with these operations. In the trial it became clear that many husbands or boyfriends had supported these women in their decision, sharing their most intimate problems. Nearly all also helped with the actual operation.[31]

## Conclusions

THERE HAS BEEN AN ATTEMPT in this paper to demonstrate the different meanings of criminal sources which can be unravelled by looking at their production to which the two parties contributed: women defendants and their judges who had quite different agenda. At the time of spectacular campaigns for abortion law reform – much celebrated in primary and secondary literature[32] – and the equally passionate counter-campaigns by opponents to reform,[33] it is easy to overlook a more important divide between official repugnance for abortion *per se* and the popular acceptance of it, especially by working-class women who regarded abortion as a solution to an undesired pregnancy. This important divide between, on the one hand, opinions publicly stated by those who determined policy, and on the other, beliefs privately held by those whose own lives were most immediately affected, was hardly noted at the time. Nor is it commented upon by historians as the main protagonists were in tacit agreement: doctors, politicians, religious spokesmen, even sex reformers and many feminists whether reformers, or not, shared a vision that the deliberate termination of pregnancy was highly problematic and could only be tolerated under the strictest regulation and medical control. Yet, for many women and their helpers, abortion was neither an act of deviance nor necessarily a tragic event. Furthermore, the aborted foetus generally was not considered a child rejected, let alone killed. It was thought of most often as a waste product, something unwanted and, therefore, to be expelled. An unwanted pregnancy was thought of as a simple misfortune that had befallen a woman, just like an illness for which a cure was needed.

As the Spitzer case showed, abortion was only one of many strategies to maintain the general well-being of a woman and her family, and so the abortionist was not seen as the dangerous and greedy quack typical of contemporary medical and political literature but somebody who could help restore the balance of the female body and of the family situation. This leads to the opening letter about Frau Spitzer and her women clients. These Berlin working-class women seemed engaged in the pursuit of domestic happiness (*häusliches Glück*) irrespective of how this was defined.[34] When it was disturbed whether by the desertion of a boyfriend or husband, the illness of a mother, the thwarted hope for a child or the fear of an unwelcome pregnancy, an appropriate remedy was sought. The fact that this could range from fortune telling to magic charms, secret potions to sympathetic magic or abortion seemed to make good sense to these women even if it seemed suspicious to the law enforcement agencies intent to control what they regarded as women's irresponsible approach to reproduction and convinced that quack abortions needed to be eradicated by all means at their disposal.

# Notes

1   In 1871, in the penal code for the newly unified Reich, abortion was deemed a criminal offence both for the pregnant woman and her accomplice, who could be punished with penal servitude for up to five years. Anybody who procured an abortion for money could be sentenced to penal servitude for up to ten years. If anybody procured an abortion without consent the sentence was to be a minimum of two years' penal servitude and if the abortion resulted in the death of the woman there was to be a minimum sentence of 10 years' penal servitude. Since 1909 there were various drafts for a new penal code which included mitigation of the penalty for the aborting woman and, from 1920 onwards, there was a powerful campaign to liberalise the law consisting of the political left, socialist physicians, feminists and sex reformers. This culminated in the law amendment of 1926 which commuted penal servitude to plain gaol for the aborting woman and her accomplice and, therefore, abortion, in this instance, was regarded no longer as a crime but as a misdemeanour tried not by a jury but by lay assessors. But for the commercial abortionist and for those who performed the abortion without consent the sentence could still be penal servitude but the maximum was now increased to 15 years. Cf. Cornelie Usborne, *The Politics of the Body in Weimar Germany. Women's reproductive rights and duties* (London & Ann Arbor, 1992), 173–4, 214–5.

2   See Usborne, *The Politics of the Body* and Atina Grossmann, *Reforming Sex* (New York & Oxford, 1995).

3   E.g. Usborne, *Politics of the Body*; Grossmann, *Reforming Sex* and Christiane Dienel, 'Das 20. Jahrhundert (I). Frauenbewegung, Klassenjustiz und das Recht auf Selbstbestimmung der Frau' in Robert Jütte (ed.), *Geschichte der Abtreibung. Von der Antike bis zur Gegenwart* (Munich, 1993), James Woycke, *Birth Control in Germany 1871–1933* (London, 1988); Kristine von Soden, 'Paragraph 218 – streichen, nicht ändern!' Abtreibung und Geburtenregelung in der Weimarer Republik' in Deutsches Hygiene Museum, Dresden (ed.), *Unter anderen Umständen. Zur Geschichte der Abtreibung* (Berlin, 1993).

4.  This paper is part of my present project to write such a 'History from Below': *The Cultures of Abortion in Weimar & Nazi Germany* (forthcoming). The history of abortion for other countries also largely centres on public discourse, see Barbara Brookes, *Abortion in England 1900–1967* (London, 1988) and Angus McLaren, *Birth Control in nineteenth-century England* (New York, 1978). Exceptions are Leslie J. Reagan, *When Abortion was a Crime. Women, Medicine, and Law in the United States, 1867–1973* (Berkeley, Los Angeles & London, 1997) and Janet Farrell Brodie, *Contraception and Abortion in 19th-century America* (Ithaca & London, 1994).

5   Cf. Usborne, *The Politics of the Body*, Ch. 4.

6   Cf. Usborne, *Politics of the Body* and her 'Abortion for sale! The competition between quacks and doctors in Weimar Germany' in Marijke Gijswijt-Hofstra, Hilary Marland and Hans de Witt (eds.), *Illness and Healing Alternatives in Western Europe* (London, 1997), 183–204. See also C. Usborne, 'Wise women, wise men and

abortion in the Weimar Republic: gender, class and medicine' in Lynn Abrams and Elizabeth Harvey (eds.), *Gender Relations in German History* (London, 1996), 143–76.

7 The German law on personal data protection requires that real names be made anonymous. All names, therefore, have been changed.

8 Landesarchiv Berlin (LAB), Rep 58, No. 2439, vol. 1, Bl. 2.

9 Cf. Detlev J.K. Peukert, *The Weimar Republic. The Crisis of Classical Modernity* (London, 1991) and Thomas W. Kniesche and Stephen Brockmann (eds.), *Dancing on the Volcano. Essays on the Culture of the Weimar Republic* (Columbia, 1994).

10 C.f. contemporary evidence in Deutscher Textilarbeiterverband (ed.), *Mein Arbeitstag, mein Wochenende. 150 Berichte von Textilarbeiterinnen* (Berlin, 1930); Irmgard Keun, *Gilgi – eine von uns* (Berlin, 1931). See also, Cornelie Usborne, 'The New Woman and generation conflict: perceptions of young women's sexual mores in the Weimar Republic' in Mark Roseman (ed.), *Generations in Conflict. Youth revolt and generation formation in Germany 1770–1968* (Cambridge, 1995), 137–63. Dagmar Reese, Eve Rosenhaft, Carola Sachse and Tilla Siegel (eds.), *Rationale Beziehungen? Geschlechterverhältnisse im Rationalisierungsprozeß* (Frankfurt a. M., 1993); Kniesche and Brockmann, *Dancing on the Volcano.*

11 Today, of course, we are used to such habits as part of the New Age movement which seems to appeal particularly, though not exclusively, to the educated middle-classes. In that sense it is obviously different from the strategies pursued by these Berlin proletarian women.

12 Cf. Mary Lindemann, *Health & Healing in Eighteenth-Century Germany* (Baltimore & London, 1996).

13 Natalie Zemon Davis, *Fiction in the Archives. Pardon Tales and their Tellers in Sixteenth-Century France* (Stanford, CA, 1987).

14 LAB, Rep 58, No. 2439, vol. 2, Bl. 175ff.

15 I.e. the Netherlands. Cf. Willem de Blécourt, 'Cultures of abortion; daily practice in The Hague, early twentieth-century' in Franz Eder, Lesley Hall and Gert Hekma (eds.), *Sexual Cultures in Europe* (Manchester, 1999).

16 LAB, Rep 58, No. 2439, vol. 1, Bl. 21–24.

17 See note 1.

18 LAB, Rep 58, No. 2439, vol. 1, Bl. 31ff.

19 Ibid., Bl. 6,31.

20 Cf. Usborne, 'Abortion for sale!', 184ff.

21 LAB, Rep 58, No. 2439, vol. 1, Bl.19.

22 Ibid., Bl. 19–20RS.

23 Regina Schulte, 'Infanticide in rural Bavaria in the nineteenth century' in Hans Medick & David Warren Sabean (eds.), *Interest and emotion. Essays on the study of family and kinship* (Cambridge, 1984), 77–102.

24  LAB, Rep 58, No. 2439, vol. 1, Bl. 21.

25  Geheimes Staatsarchiv Dahlem (GSAD), Rep 84a, Nr. 17107.

26  Ibid., Bl. 17.

27  Idem, Bl. 20.

28  Ibid., Bl. 97.

29  Ibid., Bl. 103.

30  LAB, Rep 58, No. 2439, vol. 2, Bl. 190.

31  Cf. Usborne, 'Wise women, wise men and abortion in the Weimar Republic', 143–76, 156–8.

32  E.g. The medical practitioner and writer, Carl Credé, who had been imprisoned for criminal abortion, wrote a play, *Paragraph 218, Gequälte Menschen* (Tortured people) which was staged in Berlin in 1930 by Erwin Piscator. A further famous play was written by another doctor-playwright, Friedrich Wolf, who was also accused of criminal abortion, *Cyankali*, staged in Berlin in 1929. Cf. Atina Grossmann, 'Abortion and the Economic Crisis: The 1931 Campaign against Paragraph 218' in Renate Bridenthal, Atina Grossmann and Marion Kaplan (eds.), *When Biology Became Destiny* (New York, 1984), 66–86.

33  Cf. Usborne, *The Politics of the Body*, chapter 2.

34  To restore 'domestic happiness' was indeed the promise often made in the advertisements of fortune tellers in local newspapers to attract their customers.

# 'For their own good': Drug Testing in Liverpool, West and East Africa, 1917–1938

*Helen Power*

## Introduction

IN OUR PERPETUAL QUEST to 'cope with sickness' we have been in the past, and remain today, prepared to do things that we would not otherwise consider consenting to. This includes ingesting a surprising range of foreign substances in the hope that they will cure us or make us feel better. Others whom we consider are qualified to take on this responsibility have traditionally made such decisions on our behalf.[1] In her provocative book, *Whose body is it? The troubled issue of informed consent*, Carolyn Faulder explores what she describes as the current dilemma in health care: 'the patient's right to be fully involved in making decisions' about their treatment and about their participation in experimental research.[2] The current importance of consent, particularly informed consent, in the doctor/patient relationship is a reflection of the late twentieth-century concern with autonomy as a human right: one that is brought into particularly sharp focus in the medical arena.[3] Roger Cooter writes that the ethics of the doctor/patient relationship have only recently received attention from historians. However, he considers that 'medico-social issues with present-day ethical bearings' such as human experimentation are the subject of some 'exemplary social history'.[4] This paper considers these various strands of research and argues that drug tests in the interwar period were part of the day-to-day practice and ethics of the medical encounter, at least for certain groups of patients.

The history of consent in medicine has focused on the Nuremberg Trials in the aftermath of the medical atrocities conducted by the Nazis and, to a lesser extent, the Japanese.[5] The Japanese as colonial aggressors had also engaged in human experimentation during their occupation of the Chinese mainland in the 1930s and 1940s.[6] The Nuremberg Code, established after the trials, determined that the 'voluntary consent of the human subject is absolutely essential' in medical research. The *Encyclopedia of Bioethics* informs us that 'the term "informed consent" first appeared in 1957, and serious discussion of the concept began only around 1972'.[7] Within this recent period, the early emphasis on disclosure evolved to a more complicated consideration of the 'quality of a patient's or subject's understanding of information and the right to authorise or refuse a biomedical intervention'.[8] Informed consent, therefore, is not a term that we can expect to find in sources before this period. However, this paper argues that the concept was evolving before Nuremberg. Faulder claims that, in the years following Nuremberg, the 'concept of informed consent has been extended to include medical treatment generally, that is to say clinical practice as well as clinical research'.[9] She discusses the historical antecedents of the modern term 'informed consent' as part of two discourses, one concerned with health as a human right and the other with the doctor/patient relationship. Her work continues the rather more rigorous *Human guinea pigs: Experimentation on man* by Maurice Pappworth.[10] Pappworth also questioned the acceptability of various kinds of research in clinical medicine without the prior knowledge and agreement of the patient. It is essential, nonetheless, not to transfer contemporary concerns onto historical situations. However, if it is acknowledged that the terminology is anachronistic, the idea of informed consent in day-to-day practice, as well as recognisable clinical trials, still provides a useful framework to discuss participation in research in the interwar period. Faden and Beauchamp suggest a set of criteria by which they conclude that it is possible to recognise 'an instance, practice or policy of informed consent' in any period.[11] They caution against confusing the failure to satisfy the criteria with a paucity of evidence, but admit the necessity of interpretation in assessing historical sources for evidence of informed consent.

The evolution of modern clinical trials has become a recent focus of historical investigation but, traditionally, the literature concentrates on the period after Nuremberg.[12] The pre-history of clinical trials, encompassing the experiences of rather less well organised drug testing remains relatively under-researched.[13] Post-Nuremberg it is possible to articulate such neat categories but, in the absence of an established vocabulary, it is not certain that the distinctions between patient and subject, practice and experiment were so clearly defined. Research and practice may have been overlapping activities in the minds of many practitioners if, indeed, they broke up their working day in this manner. Equally, the distinctions between patient and subject were likely to be blurred, if it is assumed the practitioner consciously considered his patient cohort in this way.[14] This is particularly the case in the testing of new drugs when manufacturers would send samples of drugs to practitioners and ask them to try the product in the normal course of treatment and provide a report. The nature of these reports was unspecified, and there was not necessarily any uniformity between different investigators who appear to have been free to experiment with methods of administration and dosage, as part of the normal therapeutic encounter.

The German dye industry had produced a range of substances useful for selective staining in histological preparations. Paul Ehrlich argued that this property could be harnessed and produce substances which 'would unite with, and destroy, the parasitic agents of disease without in any way injuring the cells of the body'.[15] His use of the word 'parasitic' did not apply only to unicellular and small multicellular organisms, however, and in the inter-war period the new synthetic drugs were most successful against tropical diseases caused by the larger parasitic organisms. The history of antiparasitic chemotherapy has received less attention than the history of antibiotics, but it provides interesting avenues for analysis. Not least because many of the new antiparasitics were toxic in therapeutic doses and had serious side effects. Much of the testing involved attempts to deal with these side effects by varying the mode of administration, size of the dose and frequency of prescription.

The race of the recipient population further complicated the clinical/experimental encounter when testing drugs in the tropics. The specific role of therapy in the history of colonial medicine has received some attention.[16] There is some useful work addressing the use of drugs by colonial regimes to combat diseases of economic importance in a subject population, apparently against their will and in stressful circumstances.[17] The prelude to widespread usage (i.e. the testing stage) awaits equal consideration, particularly with respect to the British colonies. William Bynum writes that 'historically, the socially and economically disadvantaged have always been principal subjects of human experimentation and an experimentation pattern was already well established in Hippocratic times'.[18] There is a literature on the ethics of using minority groups as experimental subjects.[19] In the case of drug tests, carried out as part of interwar tropical medicine, the subject people formed the majority, but were subject to colonial rule and the socialisation processes associated with this system of government. This is a neglected area in the history of scientific racism in medicine in general and the role of non-Caucasians as medical research subjects in particular. Wolfgang Eckart has discussed German responses to sleeping sickness in the early years of this century with particular reference to the testing of arsenical drugs. He describes the methods and motivations of physicians working in German colonies in Africa and his conclusions resonate with the issues raised in this paper.[20] The comparison of colonial experiences, with those of drug testing elsewhere during the same period, raises interesting questions. In what ways were the colonial subjects of empire used in experimentation? How does this compare with the use of prisoners, particularly in the USA;[21] research involving ethnic minorities such as the Tuskagee syphilis study;[22] or use of GPI patients for malaria research in Britain and elsewhere?[23] This paper considers some of these issues by reference to drug testing in Liverpool, West Africa and East Africa in the first half of the twentieth century. The first examples involved staff at the Liverpool School of Tropical Medicine (LSTM) and the last the Medical Department in Tanganyika Territory.

## Chemotherapy at the Liverpool School of Tropical Medicine

FROM THE EARLY YEARS OF THE CENTURY, staff at the satellite laboratory of the School in Runcorn worked on the chemotherapy of tropical diseases. Anton Breinl and Harold Wolferstan Thomas produced a reasonably useable form of atoxyl, an arsenic compound active against trypanosomiasis.[24] During the First World War, the military used the recently completed buildings of the School in Pembroke Place as a military hospital. At first dysenteric and then malarious casualties were concentrated in the wards. Both groups provided clinical material for observation and experimental therapeutics conducted by a combination of military and civilian staff, some of whom already worked for the LSTM. At the end of the war, the School revived plans to establish an overseas laboratory at Freetown in Sierra Leone. This expensive addition, funded by a legacy from the founder of the School, Sir Alfred Lewis Jones, afforded the opportunity for staff to live and work in the tropics for extended periods. In the interwar years, under the guidance of Warrington Yorke, Liverpool continued to build its reputation as a centre for chemotherapy research in the laboratory and the field and later as a centre for the training of scientific staff. In the late 1920s, the School gained support from the Medical Research Council as the MRC expanded its interests in tropical medicine and chemotherapy.[25] The School also brokered support from pharmaceutical firms to support research. In addition, at the request of a large number of drug houses in Britain and Europe, staff continued to test a range of drugs against various diseases in animal models and human patients. The overseas laboratory provided a convenient outlet for this work. Published results appeared from Liverpool and Sierra Leone and chemotherapy formed a significant part of the research culture of the LSTM at this time. The paper initially compares tests conducted during World War I, under the auspices of the military hospital located within the School, with the later tests in West Africa. Such a comparison provides a useful control for the historian: in the military cases, the racial element was missing from the possible factors that influenced the conduct of the trials.

## Anti-Malarial Work During World War I

WHEN WAR BROKE OUT IN 1914, the School offered the Tropical Ward in the Liverpool Royal Infirmary to the military authorities to provide care for tropical casualties. As soon as the new laboratory buildings of the LSTM were completed, the military also accepted the use of this space as additional hospital accommodation. Although it was under military command, the staff of the LSTM who were not on active duty worked in the hospital and enjoyed control of the two hundred beds. Ronald Ross, one time Professor of Tropical Medicine at Liverpool, but now working for the War Office in London, co-ordinated research on ways to improve the treatment of malaria. In particular, this examined the problem of relapses where, despite a presumed therapeutic dose of quinine, the patient would succumb to a repeat episode of the original infection and be rendered unfit for duty. Ross asked staff at Liverpool to utilise the clinical material to assist in this work. He took charge of the Southern and Eastern Commands, and John W.W. Stephens, Professor of Tropical Medicine, became Special Consultant for the Western, Northern and Scottish Commands. The treatment of malaria continued to rely upon a range of quinine products extracted from cinchona bark. However, the development of synthetic compounds against other diseases and new methods of laboratory investigation provided a model for a more scientific understanding of the various quinine combinations. Considerable variations in treatment schedules are in evidence in pharmacology textbooks from this period.[26] The First World War provided the means to realise a research programme by bringing together large numbers of malarious casualties at one time in circumstances that facilitated clinical research.

Soldiers infected with malaria in Macedonia and elsewhere were transferred to the military hospital at Liverpool and staff set out to 'obtain definite information, [both] clinical and microscopical of the value of certain modes of treatment' with the intention where possible 'to conduct our inquiry as to render possible a comparison of their respective values'.[27] The researchers described their ultimate aim as the elucidation of a 'curative mode of treatment'.[28] Aware that this might not be achieved, they were prepared to settle for 'detailed records of experimental work, which will have a permanent value as without such information further advance is impossible'.[29] The malarious casualties in Liverpool, over one thousand patients, represented a large cohort of experimental subjects, which could be divided into different groups to investigate methods of administration of quinine compounds and a few alternative experimental drugs. This afforded the staff at the school the chance to work out long-standing issues in malaria chemotherapy. The temporary nature of expeditions to the tropics prevented studies of any length and the facilities at the Tropical Ward in Liverpool proved no better. A diagnosis of malaria was the predominant reason for admission to the Tropical Ward of the LSTM from 1898 to the outbreak of war. However, the conditions for clinical research were far from ideal, particularly if the investigations required the prolonged hospitalisation of patients or an extended follow-up period. It was difficult to organise the individual patients in such a way that they functioned as part of a concurrent comparative study. The nature of the LSTM's relationship with the hospital authorities and those that contributed to school funds, many of whom employed the sick seamen who made up the bulk of the admissions, prevented systematic clinical research. Thus, the work was not only concerned with testing new compounds, but also with the creation of a set of baseline clinical data using existing drug regimes not previously tested comparatively on this scale. For the two years of the study, 1917–1919, for a range of treatment regimes the data recorded from these experimental investigations correlated the species of parasite treated with the relapse rate. Clinical and microscopical examinations informed the judgements on relapses. The only limiting factor was a military ruling that set a maximum of sixty days for the follow up period.

In addition to the Liverpool work, members of the team of researchers ran a shorter series of studies in Accra, on the Gold Coast (now Ghana). The aim was to measure the effectiveness of a particular treatment regime, the oral administration of a predetermined dosage of quinine sulphate in young children and adults. The Accra study attempted to replicate, as far as possible, the methodology and assessment criteria used in Liverpool. A microscopic examination of the blood determined the presence and species of malaria parasites, the blood was checked again for parasites when treatment commenced and the follow up period was set at sixty days.[30] However, there were some important differences. The numbers involved in Accra were considerably smaller than in Liverpool and it took place over a shorter period. For the most part children were the experimental subjects. They were not hospitalised, and their relapses self diagnosed or diagnosed by the parents rather than by medically qualified personnel. The aim of the tests was to determine the efficacy of a much smaller range of experimental drug regimes decided by the previous work with the adult male soldiers in Liverpool. The investigators reported that the children apparently tolerated the high oral doses of quinine sulphate. They referred to prior use of smaller doses, but had no recorded data for this part of the study. The method of administration was particularly important in Africa, 'any treatment for malaria in such subjects must be oral if it is to be favourably received by the patients themselves, their parents and their physicians'.[31] Contrary to the findings of other historians, who describe the African's acceptance of treatment that involved injections, the evidence from these studies indicates that injections were unpopular.[32] The first study in Accra involved adults as well as children. Eleven adults participated, three living in the community and eight incarcerated in the Accra asylum. The results after the initial treatment and follow-up period indicated that children relapsed whereas the adults did not. The failure to prevent relapses in the children ensured that they were potential reservoirs of infection for their community. Further work concentrated on the native children, 'with a view to obtaining further information on this matter permission was granted to examine a number of boys attending schools in Accra and to treat with quinine those found to be infected with malaria. All the boys who were thus examined were volunteers'.[33] Absence from school due to illness of an unspecified nature determined the availability of the boys for the study. Examination of the blood provided the diagnosis of malaria, but the children were not hospitalised. As 'the ages of natives in West Africa are seldom accurately known', they were arranged by their teacher in groups spanning three years to determine the effect of age upon treatment regime, relapse rate and immunity.[34] The researchers could be sure that their subjects were volunteers, but these same subjects were apparently unaware of their accurate age. Moreover, it is likely that the notion of volunteer applied to treatment rather than to participation in an experimental drug test.

Antimalarial trials with adult Europeans in Liverpool (British soldiers) and with native adults and children in Accra were concerned with establishing baseline clinical data for treatment, particularly to prevent relapses. There was no systematic involvement of adult Europeans in Accra, although there was one report of a chance observation. The goal had been to find a cure that prevented relapses, but if this could not be realised then an improved clinical picture of the treatment process would yield a series of publishable results.[35] However, this investigation involved the use of compounds in various doses that may or may not be curative. There was no concern over the issue of using sub-therapeutic doses, despite the likelihood of this causing the relapses they were working to prevent. Equally, the use of high doses in children was not questioned. None of the native patients was described as 'ill', although this had been the initial route to finding the child subjects for the second round of tests. A diagnosis of malaria was determined by blood examination looking for parasites. By contrast, the soldiers were presumably 'ill'. They were hospitalised and the series of investigations arose from the use of LSTM building as a military hospital. The work in Liverpool was at the behest of the War Office and partly funded by it. The Accra work was LSTM research and funded solely by the School. The soldiers represent experimental subjects hoping to get better. Unlike their counterparts in the experiments in West Africa, the soldiers were not described as volunteers. They were primarily patients receiving treatment. There was no discussion of consent in either the published papers or the archives dealing with the study. However, soldiers in military medical care do not have the same rights to consent as civilians since refusing treatment can be construed as disobedience and is therefore punishable. The West Africans were perceived explicitly to be taking part in a test subsumed under the rhetoric of clinical care. Some of the children in Accra may have benefited from the clinical care which the tests entailed but this was a side effect albeit a positive one.

## Later testing in West and East Africa

IN THE INTERWAR PERIOD, staff from the School repeated the style of the tests in Accra in a series of studies involving a range of other drugs. In other parts of Africa, members of the Colonial Medical Service (CMS) used their position to conduct experimental tests. Unlike the First World War antimalarial work, however, there was no directly comparable research in Britain. In the case of the LSTM, after the end of the war the military hospital closed and the buildings passed back to the LSTM. The resulting gain in laboratory facilities was matched by a diminution in the available clinical material. Later, however, for a range of drugs – 'guanidines, isothioureas, amidines and amines with alkyl and alkylene chains' – staff at the LSTM were able to use induced malaria in GPI patients to conduct unrelated experimental work out of the tropics.[36] The CMS had no such home base.

The LSTM's laboratory in Sierra Leone provided a research base in the tropics and an association with the Colonial Medical Department provided some degree of access to local people, parasites and vectors. In 1926, Rupert Gordon, Assistant Director of the Freetown laboratory, took advantage of this situation to test a new preparation of emetine against infections of *S. haematobium* in the Sierra Leone Protectorate. Before Gordon commenced his tests his colleague, Donald Blacklock, had undertaken an advisory survey for the Government and suggested public health and sanitary measures to combat schistosomiasis in the Konno district. Most of the preventative work hoped to break the cycle of transmission by environmental management and education. Blacklock discounted the use of existing preparations of emetine, i.e. the hydrochloride salt, as a means of mass treatment. The indigenous people resisted a programme involving the administration of long courses of drugs by a series of subcutaneous, intramuscular or intravenous injections. Only in circumstances that permitted hospitalisation could the value of this drug be realised: in rural Sierra Leone, this was impracticable. The Government Medical Department assisted the tests by providing Gordon with a grant for travelling expenses. The United Brethren in Christ Mission School provided the experimental subjects, and Miss E. Grant from the United Brethren in Christ Mission Hospital at Jiama, Nimmi Korro helped carry out the 'courses of treatment'.[37] Dr W. Martindale of Martindale Chemists, who prepared and described the drug, supplied the samples used in the tests, via his connections with Warrington Yorke in Liverpool.[38] Gordon explained the rationale behind his programme of research:

> The West African native, although objecting strongly to all forms of injection does not appear to extend this prejudice to medicines taken by mouth and will travel great distances to report daily for longer periods in order to obtain drugs of this description. It appears clear therefore that any drug capable of curing schistosomiasis by oral administration will prove of very great value in the tropics, both for the treatment of individual cases and still more so for the mass treatment of intensely infected areas where the drug can be distributed by a native dispenser without incurring the risks associated with the giving of subcutaneous injections by an unqualified person.[39]

He justified its experimental nature in terms of the benefits likely to accrue to the community at large should the drug prove efficacious. Thus, the people of the Korro region were being used to test a preparation that could benefit their fellow colonial subjects, however, their individual involvement was to be interpreted as a therapeutic encounter. The subjects of the study were 81 children examined at the United Brethren in Christ Missionary School. Of the 81, 43 had evidence of *S. haematobium* in the bladder. Of these, 28 were classified as severe cases, i.e. they were passing live eggs and blood in every sample of urine examined. The 28 severe cases were divided into two groups of 14. The first received subcutaneous injections of emetine hydrochloride as a control and the second group were given emetine periodide by mouth. Microscopical examination of the children's urine on alternate days during treatment, and for eight days after the end of the treatment period, provided the means to assess the relative efficacy of these drugs and methods of administration. The researchers reported 'considerable difficulty ... in making the children attend for their injections and disciplinary action had to be taken to ensure that each child completed its full course'.[40] This is perhaps unsurprising given the side effects: there were several cases of 'emetine nodules' and 'sore arms' after fifteen days of consecutive injections. The most severe case involved a child who 'four days after the completion of his treatment, developed some rather alarming signs of heart failure which disappeared after two days rest in bed'.[41] The results of the use of emetine periodide were more encouraging. Gordon took the drug out of its gelatine capsule and gave the powder in milk. He reported that 'no unpleasant symptoms such as those recorded with the use of emetine hydrochloride followed the taking of emetine periodide by mouth and it is important to note that no difficulty whatsoever was experienced in getting the children to report for, and take, their medicine'.[42] Gordon considered the test a resounding success. He acknowledged that among those cured there might be cases of relapse in the future. He cautioned, however, that in an endemic area it was difficult to judge if relapses were real or cases of re-infection. He noted that this issue required more careful study than circumstances permitted. In the absence of all unpleasant symptoms, he proposed the use of larger doses. The use of the African children in this way required no particular justification. Gordon, the staff of the school and hospital at Korro and the Colonial Government, who subsidised the tests, regarded it as legitimate in light of the prevailing conditions of ill health. In effect, they considered they were offering treatment to children who would otherwise have been unlikely to receive such clinical care. It is symptomatic of the paternalist attitude of colonial medicine that the researchers failed to perceive the need to inform the children, or their parents, of either the nature of their immediate activities (the experimental use of new drugs), or the potential of the work (the long term benefit to the community).

As the opportunity arose, LSTM staff and others continued to test new drugs in Africa in the later 1920s and 1930s. In Liverpool, the increasing concentration of research activities in the field of chemotherapy provided increased contact with drug companies. The creation of two committees by the MRC and Colonial Office in 1927 and 1936, concerned with research in colonial and tropical medicine, and the MRC's continued interest in chemotherapy, through the Chemotherapy Committee, stimulated additional research.[43] The increased financial support and the interest of the colonial authorities coincided with a more proactive use of colonial subjects in drug tests. By the late 1930s, researchers no longer subsumed their tests under the rubric of clinical practice and turned to the open use of Africans in non-therapeutic drug tests, involving the direct infection of experimental subjects with parasites. From the mid-1920s, J.F. Corson, Medical Officer of the Tinde Laboratory, and his colleague, Professor F.K. Kleine, were involved with experimental treatment of sleeping sickness patients using Bayer 205 (germanin), Tryparsamide and BR 68 at the Ikoma hospital in Tanganyika Territory.[44] Kleine was a member of the League of Nations International Committee on Human Trypanosomiasis and the work at Ikoma contributed to the deliberations of that committee.[45] The tests involved variations in the size of doses and observation of the effects of giving these drugs alone or in combination. The goal was to achieve sterilisation of the cerebro-spinal fluid after using lumber punctures to detect the presence and then the absence of trypanosomes. The continued absence of parasites would ensure that the patient did not suffer a relapse and that the case was described as a cure.[46] As in the anti-schistosomiasis trials, researchers indicated the difficulties of ensuring that patients would attend for treatment that involved a prolonged series of injections.[47] Manipulation of dosage and method of administration was therefore an important element in these tests. In 1938, using his experience of treating 'thousands of cases' with Bayer 205, Corson sought to recruit African volunteers for a series of tests involving the experimental infection with *T. rhodesiense*, one of the parasites responsible for sleeping sickness (human trypanosomaisis). The necessity of experimental over naturally acquired infections is unclear from the paper, although he refers twice to the importance of the work in the preamble. The majority of the publication is concerned with legitimising the use of human subjects to determine the side effects of a particular dosage and method of administering the drug. He opened the discussion by cautioning against the indiscriminate use of Africans as voluntary experimental subjects when the test lacked the obvious therapeutic benefits. He neglected to refer to the side effect of blindness that frequently accompanied the use of Bayer 205 when stressing the benefits of the previous tests. He referred instead to the subordinate racial position of the Africans in the colonial encounter; the paternalism of the Europeans, which could act as sufficient safeguard for research of this kind; and the informed decision that the Africans had taken in agreeing to participate:

> It will be generally agreed that unsophisticated African volunteers should not be used for experimental infection with *Trypanosoma rhodesiense* unless the experimenter is convinced, on good grounds, that the infection will be free from risk of permanent injury to the health of volunteers. Natives can at least understand, even if they cannot estimate, such risks as hunting dangerous animals or swimming flooded rivers, which they may undertake in the service of white people; these are risks which form part of their ordinary life. As regards infection with *T. rhodesiense* the volunteers mentioned in this record had seen others resist infection or recover from it, or had been told about it by them; they knew that the bite of the infective fly might be followed by local swelling and fever, and they accepted my assurance, or that of former volunteers that the experiment was safe. They had sufficient intelligence and experience of Europeans to believe that such an experiment would not be made without a sure remedy for the disease. In fact, it may be said that they had some evidence and knowledge to guide them in deciding to offer themselves as volunteers.[48]

Corson continued his discussion of the research methodology with reference to the use of European volunteers:

> I have to acknowledge the offers of a few European men and women to be volunteers; it could not reasonably be expected, however, that many residents in tropical Africa would be sufficiently interested or sufficiently free to interrupt their duties and to allow themselves to undergo the discomfort of an attack of sleeping sickness and its treatment. It seems, then, that when the experiments are sufficiently important, the use of African volunteers is justified.[49]

The comment that Europeans were insufficiently interested in the development of an effective treatment against sleeping sickness is revealing. It is perhaps indicative of the confidence attached to the use of Bayer 205, providing it was administered sufficiently early in the infection and in an appropriately large dose, circumstances most easily achieved by Europeans. Such knowledge had been gained over the course of several years by using African patients who were often caught in an epidemic of the disease. Moreover, the busy lives of Europeans that prevented their experimental infection with trypanosomiasis reinforces the racial divide in colonial medicine. After wading through Corson's polemic, the real reason for the Africans' volunteering becomes apparent:

> It was thought unwise, and was found to be unnecessary, to use any persuasion or any form of propaganda to induce volunteers to present themselves ... a relatively large reward of money, however, was offered and their motive in volunteering was, of course, to gain it. They showed and expressed pleasure when an official appreciation of their action was conveyed to them.[50]

During the tests, Corson listed the main side effect of administering the drug as albuminuria resulting from kidney damage. Previous papers describing the experimental use of Bayer 205 referred to the potential severity of this condition, particularly when larger doses were used.[51] Here, he expressed concern only if this condition should appear early in the treatment. In reviewing the results, he dismissed this serious side effect and other minor ones with comparative ease:

> There was no reason to think that either the infections with trypanosomes or the treatment with germanin had anything to so with the complications, except with the albuminuria ... There seems to be no reason to think that ... intercurrent illnesses were exceptional among these people, who are expressed to many parasitic diseases, have primitive ideas about health and sanitation, and are mostly careless and thoughtless. Puzzling illnesses are commonly ascribed to witchcraft. The more serious complications fortunately occurred after the 3rd or 4th dose of germanin had been given so that the infection with trypanosomes could be regarded as cured before the complication appeared.[52]

Particularly revealing is the faith that the researchers expressed in the African's ability to make an informed judgement on their participation in the test, and yet they are equally vociferous in their denigration of the African's belief in witchcraft. On the one hand, they treat them as intelligent adults, on the other they regard them as superstitious children. If statements such as this reinforce our understanding of the relationships of the colonial encounter, what can they tell us of their use as experimental subjects? It was acceptable that Africans, as a group, were to benefit from research in which some of their number not only participated as passive patients, but as active experimental subjects. Under the benevolence of their colonial overlords, selected Africans were obliged to accept a role that enabled their wider community to benefit from western medicine as introduced by the colonial practitioners.

## Conclusion

THIS PAPER BRINGS TOGETHER elements of the histories of human experimentation, clinical practice, colonialism and tropical medicine in the interwar years. It has addressed some of the ways in which the colonial encounter between European doctors and indigenous patients can be incorporated into the already complicated analyses of consent. The evolution of protocols for clinical trials aimed to better the standards of scientific investigation and protect the participants. Formal rules, ensuring the provision of adequate information concerning the potential risks to the participant and the need to gain their voluntary agreement to take part in a clinical trial, replaced the ad hoc personal judgements of acceptable practice as seen here.

The criteria that Faden and Beauchamp consider potentially detectable before this time, proved difficult to put into practice in interwar colonial medicine because of pre-existing social and cultural patterns. These patterns based on inequalities in the medical and colonial encounters make it difficult to conceive that adequate consent could be achieved. The subjects were of a different class from the practitioner; many were of a different gender; many were minors; the majority were already sick and/or dying; all were of a different race from the practitioner and part of a colonised population. In the tests reviewed here, the decision that it was in the interest of the patient to become a test participant was made for them, as this course of action was deemed to be in that individual's best interest. Certainly not all knew they were in effect experimental subjects. Such attitudes were prevalent in the general delivery of health care in the colonial situation, which routinely involved drug tests. However, there is an awareness that as the tests become overtly experimental, the principle of consent became more important, but the use of human subjects, despite their inferior position, was still accepted as necessary.

In the period before the advent of protocols, much clinical research was in fact part of day-to-day clinical practice and patient care.[53] There was not necessarily a clear distinction between what constituted clinical practice and clinical research. We would regard the testing of drugs as experiments: an innovative procedure with no established outcome. In the 1930s, the legal definition of an experiment in medicine referred to a departure from standard medical practice. In the work cited in this paper, standard medical practice routinely involved the use of new substances, and variations in their dosage and method of administration. This may explain why practitioners did not consider that they were experimenting as such. Indeed, the issue was raised only when the African subjects were deliberately infected rather than behaving as the passive recipients of western medicine. In the 1930s, it was argued that the indigenous population of the African colonies could expect access to health and welfare provision from the colonial government. Ironically, this right brought with it a permissive attitude to the use of Africans in practices deemed to be for their own good.

It is possible to distinguish three levels among experiments performed in clinical medicine: experiments done for the possible direct benefit of the patient/subject; experiments done which are likely to be of benefit to a class of individuals with which the subjects identify; experiments which have no direct benefit to the subjects taking part. The tests in Liverpool, Accra and Korro fall into the first two categories. The tests in Tanganyika had no direct benefit for the participants, but the researchers assumed on their behalf that the results would be useful to other Africans. It would be convenient given the evidence described above to argue that this was because of their perceived racial inferiority. The evidence from the work in Liverpool in the First World War and similar work in World War II muddies this picture.[54] There was little more regard for the British soldiers than their African counterparts. These examples indicate that drug testing, in the era before patient autonomy replaced the beneficence model of medicine, is as much about the perceptions of the day-to-day doctor/patient encounter as well as special studies of experimental medicine.

# Notes

1    J. Katz, *The Silent World of Doctor and Patient* (New York & London, 1984).

2    C. Faulder, *Whose Body Is It? The Troubling Issue of Informed Consent* (London, 1985), p.1.

3    M.J. Franzblau, 'Ethical Values in Health Care in 1995: Lessons from the Nazi Period', *Journal of the Medical Association of Georgia*, 84 (1995), 161–4; A. Goldworth, 'Informed Consent in the Human Genome Enterprise', *Cambridge Quarterly of Healthcare Ethics*, 4 (1995), 296–303; N.E. Brazell, 'The Significance and Application of Informed Consent', *AORN Journal*, 65 (1997) 377–80, 382, 385–6.

4    R. Cooter, 'The Resistible Rise of Medical Ethics', *Social History of Medicine*, 8 (1995), 257–70, p. 257.

5    G.J. Annas, *The Nazi Doctors and the Nuremberg Code: Human Rights in Human Experimentation* (New York, 1992).

6    T. Brnighausen, *Medizinische Humanexperimente der japanischen Truppen für Biologische Kriegsfhrung in China, 1932–1945* (Diss. med., Med. Fak. Univ. Heidelberg, 1996).

7    W.T. Reich (ed.), *Encyclopedia of Bioethics* (revised edition, New York, 1995), 3, p. 1232.

8    Ibid.

9    Faulder, *Whose Body Is It?*, pp. 12–3.

10   M.H. Pappworth, *Human Guinea Pigs: Experimentation on Man* (London, 1967).

11   R. Faden & T. Beauchamp, *A History and Theory of Informed Consent* (New York, 1986), p. 54.

12   For example, see B.H. Gray, *Human Subjects in Medical Experimentation: A Sociological Study of the Conduct and Regulation of Clinical Research* (New York, 1975); P.M. McNeill, *The Ethics and Politics of Human Experimentation* (Cambridge, 1993).

13   J. Vollman & R. Winau, 'Informed Consent in Human Experimentation Before the Nuremberg Code', *British Medical Journal*, 313 (1996), 1445–7; D. Cox-Maksimov, *The Making of the Clinical Trial in Britain, 1910–1945: Expertise, the State and the Public* (unpublished PhD thesis, University of Cambridge, 1997).

14   How patients/subjects classified their experiences is even more difficult to determine.

15   R.J. Schnitzer & F. Hawking, *Experimental chemotherapy* (New York, 1963) 1, p. 3.

16   J.M. Janzen, *The Quest for Therapy in Lower Zaire* (Berkeley, 1978); M. Vaughan, *Curing Their Ills: Colonial Power and African Illness* (Cambridge, 1991); L. White, '"They Could Make Their Victims Dull": Genders and Genres, Fantasies and Cures in Colonial Southern Uganda', *American Historical Review*, (1995), 1379–1402. I am grateful to Marisa Chambers for drawing my attention to this reference.

17  *Proceedings of the First International Conference on Sleeping Sickness, London 17th of June 1907*, London HMSO, 1907 cd3778; M. Lyons, 'Death Camps in the Congo: Administrative Responses to Sleeping Sickness, 1903–11', *Bulletin Society Social History of Medicine*, 34 (1984), 28–31.

18  W. Bynum, 'Reflections on the History of Human Experimentation' in S.F. Spicker et al. (eds.), *The Use of Human Beings in Research with Special Reference to Clinical Trials* (Dordrecht, Boston & London, 1988), pp. 29–46, p. 32. See also B. Elkeles, 'Medizinische Menschenversuche gegen Ende des 19. Jahrhunderts und der Fall Neisser. Rechtfertigung und Kritik einer wissenschaftlichen Methode', *Medizinhistorisches Journal*, 20 (1985), 135–48. I am grateful to Wolfgang Eckart for this reference.

19  C.R. McCarthy, 'Historical Background of Clinical Trials Involving Women and Minorities', *Academic Medicine*, 69 (1994), 695–701; J.H. Jones, *Bad Blood: The Tuskegee Syphilis Experiment* (New York, 1993); T.L. Savitt, 'The Use of Blacks for Medical Experimentation and Demonstration in the Old South', *Journal of Southern History*, XLVIII (1982), 331–48.

20  W.U. Eckart, 'The Colony as Laboratory and the Fight against Sleeping Sickness in German East Africa and Togo' (forthcoming, 1999).

21  A.M. Hornblum, 'They Were Cheap and Available: Prisoners as Research Subjects in Twentieth Century America', *British Medical Journal*, 315 (ii) (1997), 1437–41; J.M. Harkness, 'Prisoners and Pellagra', *Public Health Reports*, 111 (1996), 463–7.

22  A.M. Brandt, 'Racism and Research: The Case of the Tuskagee Syphilis Study' in J.W. Leavitt & R.L. Numbers, *Sickness and Health in America* (Madison & London, 1985) pp. 331–46.

23  H.R. Rollin, 'The Horton Malaria Laboratory, Epsom, Surrey (1925–1975)', *Journal of Medical Biography*, 2 (1994), 94–7.

24  H.W. Thomas, 'The Experimental Treatment of Trypanosomiasis in Animals', *Proceedings of the Royal Society, Series B*, LXXVI (1905), 589–91.

25  H.J. Power, *Tropical Medicine in the Twentieth Century: A History of the Liverpool School of Tropical Medicine, 1898–1990* (London, 1999).

26  L. Rogers, *Fevers in the Tropics* (Calcutta, 1907); A.R. Cushney, *A Textbook of Pharmacology and Therapeutics: Or the Action of Drugs in Health and Disease* (London, 1910); W.H. Martindale, *The Extra Pharmacopoeia* (London, 1915); A.J. Clark, *Applied Pharmacology* (London, 1937).

27  J.W.W. Stephens, W. Yorke, B. Blacklock, J.W.S. Macfie & C.F. Cooper, 'Studies in the Treatment of Malaria', *Annals of Tropical Medicine and Parasitology*, 11 (1917–18), 91–111, p. 92.

28  Ibid.

29  Ibid.

30  J.W. Macfie & M.W. Fraser, 'Oral Administration of Quinine or Quinine and Arsenic for Short Periods to Young Native Children Infected with Malignant

Tertian Malaria', *Annals of Tropical Medicine and Parasitology*, 14 (1920–21), 83–91; J.W.S. Macfie, 'Oral Administration of Quinine Sulphate Grains 20 to Adult Natives Infected with Malignant Tertian Malaria', *Annals of Tropical Medicine and Parasitology*, 14 (1920–21), 93–4.

31  Macfie & Fraser, 'Oral Administration of Quinine or Quinine and Arsenic', 91.

32  White, '"They Could Make Their Victims Dull"', p. 1392.

33  J.W.S. Macfie, 'Oral Administration of Quinine Sulphate Grains 10 Daily for 2 Consecutive Days Only for Native School-boys Infected with Malignant Tertian Malaria', *Annals of Tropical Medicine and Parasitology*, 14 (1920–21), 95–109, p 95.

34  Ibid.

35  J.W.W. Stephens, 'Studies in the Treatment of Malaria XXXII: Summary of Studies I–XXXI', *Annals of Tropical Medicine and Parasitology*, 17 (1923), 303–5.

36  F. Glyn-Hughes, E.M. Lourie & W. Yorke, 'Studies in Chemotherapy XVII: The Action of Undecane Diamidine in Malaria', *Annals of Tropical Medicine and Parasitology*, 32 (1938), 103–7, p. 103.

37  R.M. Gordon, 'Emetine Periodide in the Treatment of *S. heamatobium* Infections Among West African Children', *Annals of Tropical Medicine and Parasitology*, 20 (1926), 229–37, p. 236.

38  W.H. Martindale, 'A Note on Emetine Preparation for Rectal and Oral Use', *Transactions of the Royal Society of Tropical Medicine and Hygiene*, XVII (1923), 27–32.

39  Gordon, 'Emetine Periodide in the Treatment of *S. heamatobium*', p. 230.

40  Ibid., p. 236.

41  Ibid., p. 234.

42  Ibid.

43  J. Beinart, 'The Inner World of Imperial Sickness: The MRC and Research in Tropical Medicine' in J. Austoker & L. Bryder (eds.), *Historical Perspectives on the Role of the MRC* (Oxford, 1989), pp. 109–35.

44  J.F. Corson, 'Sleeping Sickness in the Ikoma District of Tanganyika Territory: Notes on Some Cases Treated by Professor F.K. Kleine', *Annals of Tropical Medicine and Parasitology*, 22 (1928), 379–418.

45  F.K. Kleine, 'Report on the New Sleeping Sickness Focus at Ikoma', *Final Report of the League of Nations International Committee on Human Trypanosomiasis*, 1928.

46  G. Maclean & H. Fairburn, 'Treatment of Rhodesian Sleeping Sickness with Bayer 205 and Tryparasimide: Observations on 719 Cases', *Annals of Tropical Medicine and Parasitology*, 26 (1932), 157–89.

47  Maclean & Fairburn, 'Treatment of Rhodesian Sleeping Sickness with Bayer 205', p. 161.

48  J.F. Corson, 'A record of some complications which occurred in the course of experimental infections of African volunteers with *Trypanosoma rhodesiense*', *Annals of Tropical Medicine and Parasitology*, 32 (1938), 437–43, p. 437.

49  Ibid., p. 439.

50  Ibid.

51  Maclean & Fairburn, 'Treatment of Rhodesian Sleeping Sickness with Bayer 205', p. 175.

52  Ibid., pp. 442–3.

53  D. Weatherall, *Medicine and the Quiet Art: Medical Research and Patient Care* (Oxford, 1995).

54  H.J. Power, 'Malaria, Drugs and World War II', paper presented 6 May 1994, *Malaria & War symposium*, Wellcome Institute for the History of Medicine, London.

# Law, Medicine and Morality: A Comparative View of Twentieth-Century Sexually Transmitted Disease Controls

*Roger Davidson & Lutz D.H. Sauerteig*

## Introduction

ONE OF THE MORE CONTENTIOUS INTERFACES between the law and medicine in the last 150 years has been the response of civil society to infectious and contagious diseases, and none more so than in its response to Venereal Disease (VD) and other Sexually Transmitted Diseases (STDs). By the early twentieth century, VD had become in many countries a metaphor for physical and moral decay and for the forces of pollution and contamination that appeared to threaten social order and racial progress. Alarm over the issue of VD reflected broader concerns over the moral direction of society, and its supposedly wilful nature and threat to social hygiene provided a powerful justification for the social construction and regulation of 'dangerous sexualities'.[1]

The debate over VD raised, and indeed still continues to raise, a range of fundamental and contentious issues relating to the use of legal compulsion for the purposes of disease control, and the appropriate balance within policy-making between the interests of public health and the liberty of the individual. It has also provoked extensive discussion as to the relationship of the law to morality and sexuality, and to the discriminatory features often implicit in that relationship in terms of class, gender and race. What is striking from the growing literature on the social history of VD around the world is the variety of outcomes to this discourse. Some countries have adopted what might be termed coercive strategies within which the law has been extensively mobilised to regulate the infected and to penalise the wilful neglect of treatment or spread of disease, while at the other end of the spectrum, there are countries whose public health strategies can be broadly defined as voluntaristic, with an emphasis on free and accessible treatment and health education.[2] This study seeks to explore some of the variables that have shaped this variance by reference to the German and Scottish experiences, and their variance from the ideology and practice of policy in England.[3]

## Germany

IN BOTH GERMANY AND ENGLAND at the turn of the century, the issue arose in medical debate as to what extent VD should be treated under public health legislation in line with other infectious diseases. In particular, it was debated whether VD should be compulsorily notifiable and whether those infected should be legally obliged to seek qualified treatment and be forced to undergo treatment even against their will. Similar arguments for and against the compulsory notification of VD prevailed in both countries. The main argument in favour of compulsory notification was that only notification would ensure proper treatment for those who refused to comply with medical advice and who thus endangered public health. The main argument against compulsory notification from the viewpoint both of German and British physicians was that the confidentiality between doctor and patient would be undermined. Furthermore, compulsion would lead to concealment of infection and thus would drive patients to resort to lay healers. In general, especially in England, compulsory methods were considered to be an infringement of the citizen's liberty.[4]

In Prussia, in the aftermath of the Napoleonic wars, compulsory notification for syphilis was first introduced in a Public Health Act of 1835, but doctors virtually ignored this provision.[5] However, the experience of coping with a devastating cholera epidemic that swept through the German harbour town of Hamburg in 1892 provoked a fresh review of infectious diseases legislation.[6] An Imperial Act of 1900 introduced compulsory notification for certain infectious diseases.[7] Members of the German women's movement, in their struggle for abolition of the State regulation of prostitution, were in favour of including VD in this Act.[8] They argued that, by introducing general compulsory notification, not only the prostitute but also her male client would have to be reported as a threat to the health of other women. In the event, many areas of the medical profession and the public health administration strongly rejected this idea and VD could not be brought under this act.

Likewise, the Catholic Centre Party did not succeed in introducing legislation to penalise a person with VD who exposed his or her sexual partner to the risk of infection.[9] Leading law experts such as the Berlin penologist, Franz von Liszt, and venereologists like Albert Neisser, Professor in Breslau, also demanded a tightening of the penal law in this direction. Von Liszt was convinced that, because of its educational value and deterrent effect, such a reform would help to prevent non-marital sexual relations.[10] Other law experts considered the existing regulations of the German Penal Law as sufficient. Under the Penal Law, the deliberate and wilful communication of any infectious disease was already indictable as an assault. Yet, it was very difficult to prove this in a case of VD and cases involving a sentence of imprisonment were exceptional.[11] However, under new proposals, it was intended not only to penalise the wilful transmission of VD but also any exposure to a possible risk of infection. Thus, it would have been unnecessary to prove that venereal infection had actually taken place as a result of a specific sexual contact.

Finally, the emergency situation of the First World War fostered a greater willingness to introduce more radical steps towards combating VD. Under emergency legislation of 1918, a person could be convicted of assault when he or she endangered a sexual partner with a venereal infection. The maximum penalty was three years imprisonment.[12] This legislation was strongly supported by members of the women's movement, some leading law experts, and venereologists such as Albert Neisser and Alfred Blaschko, both from the German Society for Combating VD (*Deutsche Gesellschaft zur Bekämpfung der Geschlechtskrankheiten*).[13] It should be noted that, in the 1920s, an average of about 650 people per year, seventy-five per cent of them women, were convicted under this legislation. However, none incurred the possible maximum penalty, with the majority sentenced to less than three months imprisonment.[14] In addition, there were proposals for the compulsory notification of soldiers with VD. Following their discharge from the military, such soldiers were to be reported to the Social Insurance Boards for supervision of further treatment. However, since the military was opposed to compulsory measures, this procedure remained voluntarily and thus only rarely used.[15]

True compulsion was eventually introduced under the 1927 German Act for Combating VD. It required everyone with VD to be treated by a qualified doctor, and medical practitioners were compelled to notify health authorities of any patient who failed to comply with their treatment regimes, who defaulted from treatment, or who continued to endanger public health by remaining sexually active despite being infected. The health authorities could then commit these patients for further treatment to the lock-ward of a hospital, using police force if necessary.[16] The 1927 Act, which is still in force today, albeit with some modifications,[17] was a critical point in the long German tradition of State intervention in VD control. After intense debates about the relationship of personal liberty to public health controls, a definite decision in favour of the public interest had been made. This policy was supported by the influential German Society for Combating VD and by public health administrators, such as the President of the Imperial Social Insurance Office. Thus, the Chairman of the Society for Combating VD, the venereologist Joseph Jadassohn, declared in the *Reichstag* (the German Parliament) in 1923, 'Personal rights stop where they compete with the welfare of the public.'[18] There was a broad party consensus that VD patients had a responsibility towards the family, the future of the State and the race. The State, therefore, had the right to force a VD patient to be treated. However, there was no overwhelming consensus in favour of general compulsory notification for VD. Many doctors strongly advised against such proposals as they were afraid that they might undermine the fundamental ethics of confidentiality.[19]

The 1927 VD Act substantially extended medical controls. Under the Act, it was not only the prostitute who was under medical control but her male client as well. Thus, whereas in England the Contagious Diseases Acts, passed by Parliament in the 1860s to control the spread of VD in the military by introducing compulsory diagnosis, treatment and police registration of women suspected of being prostitutes, were repealed in 1886,[20] the German VD Act of 1927 functioned as a substitute for the State regulation of prostitution which had been in force up to that time. The vice squads of the police were abolished and their role was taken over by doctors and the health administration.[21]

## England

MEANWHILE, IN ENGLAND, the tendency was in the other direction. In 1912, the Local Government Board, which was responsible for public health policy, asked one of its senior medical inspectors, Ralph W.

Johnstone, to conduct an investigation of the prevalence and treatment of VD in England. In his report, Johnstone came to the conclusion that 'the best method of controlling venereal diseases and protecting the free from infection would be the provision of means for early and accurate diagnosis, with skilled advice and adequate treatment available for all infected persons'. Johnstone clearly rejected any form of notification, for which he considered the time not yet to be ripe, as well as compulsory detention for treatment which, he argued, would 'defeat its own end'.[22]

This influential report became the basis of a voluntaristic approach to VD controls. The Medical Officer of the Local Government Board, Arthur Newsholme, concurred with Johnstone's conclusions. In his view, notification would 'tend to concealment of disease and delay in or neglect of skilled treatment'.[23] In its 1916 report, the Royal Commission on Venereal Diseases, of which Arthur Newsholme was a member, also advised against introducing compulsory notification or compulsory continuance of treatment. The commissioners feared that compulsion would deter infected persons from seeking qualified treatment at the earliest possible moment. Instead, the Royal Commission recommended on the one hand that the government should extend confidential and free diagnostic and treatment facilities, and on the other, that it should educate the public on the grave dangers arising from VD.[24] The Local Government Board incorporated most of these suggestions in its 1916 VD Regulations.[25] Under these regulations, a new health service system of treatment centres was to be established, two-thirds of the funding coming from the Exchequer and one-third from local taxation. By December 1920, local authorities in England and Wales had opened up 185 treatment centres. By 1925, their number had increased by nine, and by 1930, 189 treatment centres were open to the public. At these treatment centres, anyone could obtain information along with free and confidential examination and treatment, when appropriate. The treatment centres were an important step for Britain in setting up a comprehensive government-funded public health system.[26]

Furthermore, a National Council for Combating VD (NCCVD) was founded in 1914 with the aim of educating the public on VD. For this purpose, the NCCVD obtained financial support from the Local Government Board and later the Ministry of Health as well as from local authorities. During the 1920s, the NCCVD functioned as a semi-official organisation to co-ordinate all public health activities dealing with the 'propaganda' aspects of VD. In its health education campaigns, the NCCVD spread information on the horrible symptoms of VD and recommended chastity and sexual self-control as the best way of preventing infection.

Hence, the main aim of the NCCVD was moral education. In cases where moral education had failed and venereal infection was contracted, the NCCVD strongly recommended those infected to seek qualified treatment immediately.[27]

The subsequent history of VD policy in England certainly featured a number of debates over the issue of compulsion, but it was essentially a story of the repeated triumph of voluntarism over the forces of coercion. The Royal Commission on VD had anticipated that the issue of legal controls might have to be reconsidered at some future date.[28] However, even faced with the wartime escalation in the incidence of VD among British soldiers, the British government stuck to the principle of voluntarism and concentrated on the provision of treatment centres and propaganda to encourage the public to seek prompt and professional advice. Pressed by the Dominions, the Home Secretary, Sir George Cave, did introduce in February 1917 a Criminal Law Amendment Bill penalising those who were infected who had intercourse or who solicited intercourse, and requiring offenders to undergo compulsory medical examination. Opposition, especially from the women's movement and social purity organisations, successfully aborted the bill but, in March 1918, the War Cabinet eventually approved a Defence of the Realm Regulation (DORA) 40D making it a criminal offence for women infected with VD to solicit or have sexual relations with members of His Majesty's forces. This coercive measure enjoyed only half-hearted support even from the War Cabinet and Home Office. During the seven months of its operation, 201 women were prosecuted and 102 convicted under DORA 40D. Again, a storm of protest came from the women's movement and social purity organisations who viewed the new regulation as an attempt to reintroduce the much hated Contagious Diseases Acts. The regulation was duly withdrawn at the end of the war.[29]

Again, in the 1920s, some venereologists, such as the Secretary General of the Society for the Prevention of Venereal Diseases, Hugh Wansy Bayly, many Medical Officers of Health, and a range of local authorities advocated stricter controls of VD patients, and particularly of defaulters who discontinued their treatment prematurely and represented both a waste of public funds and a risk to public health.[30] At the beginning of the 1920s, the position of the influential NCCVD regarding the question of compulsory notification and treatment was ambivalent. A minority of members seem to have favoured some form of compulsion. For example, the NCCVD's Medical Secretary, Otto May, argued, that 'If "liberty of the subject" is to mean "liberty to spread disease without hindrance", then the sooner such liberty is destroyed, the better for civilisation!'[31] The majority, however, was hesitant, and in 1920 the Executive Committee of the NCCVD agreed that they '[did] not at present advocate the adoption of a system of general compulsory notification of Venereal Disease' but intended to submit a draft bill designed 'to secure the continuous treatment of infected persons' sometime in the future when public opinion demanded such a regulation.[32] In 1922, the NCCVD devoted a whole issue of its journal, *Health & Empire*, to the question of notification in order to stimulate the ongoing debate over how to regulate defaulting patients,[33] but the issue of compulsion was subsequently overshadowed by the controversy surrounding VD prophylaxis.[34]

In the late 1920s and the 1930s, the advocates of compulsion renewed their campaign within several branches of the NCCVD, renamed the British Social Hygiene Council (BSHC) in 1925.[35] For example, Charles J. Bond, the former Chairman of the Leicester Branch of the NCCVD and Vice-Chairman on Lord Dawson's Council on Medical and Allied Services, an advisory body to the Minister of Health, argued in 1926 in favour of increasing the sense of individual responsibility towards a healthy citizenship. Bond was convinced that 'the time has come to re-estimate and revalue our judgements concerning secrecy in all relations of life. We must be willing to relinquish some of our cherished so-called individual rights, in order to obtain a healthier communal life.' Consequently, he wanted to have VD included in the list of notifiable diseases with penal consequences for infected persons who failed to obtain or continue treatment and who knowingly transmitted their infection.[36] Similarly, the VD Officer for the City of Salford, E.T. Burke, tried to demonstrate in 1935 that a large majority of his patients were willing to accept compulsory treatment.[37] However, the Executive Committee of the BSHC agreed in February 1932, 'that the present was not a very suitable time to press for increased powers'.[38] In an editorial, entitled 'A Threat of Compulsion!', *Health & Empire* depicted the 'voluntary character of the British Venereal Diseases Scheme' as being 'in line with British tradition, which puts great stress on personal liberty'.[39] Yet, as Sir Basil Blackett stressed in his presidential address to the Council in July 1935, the voluntary principle in VD control 'impose[d] its own responsibilities' for the individual as well as for health services, a fact, he claimed, that was not yet fully appreciated.[40] Thus, what was necessary to solve current shortcomings and defects in the VD system was not compulsion but continuous public health education 'to meet the conditions of prejudice and of general ignorance'.[41]

The Ministry of Health refused to support any form of compulsory notification or treatment in the 1920s and 1930s. It considered that the existing VD policy of free and confidential treatment was more effective than any coercive measure. Compulsion was still regarded as an unjustified invasion of the privacy of the citizen.[42] The policy of the Ministry of Health was supported by a semi-official Committee on VD, installed by Sir Alfred Mond, the Minister of Health, in 1922. Lord Trevethin, the former Chief Justice, was appointed as Chairman; the majority of the Committee's members were physicians, including Charles Bond. In its report, the Trevethin Committee rejected compulsory notification as useless if not supported by a system of compulsory treatment. This, they argued, would only lead to concealment, deter infected persons from treatment, and be detrimental to existing VD policy. Moreover, the Committee came to the conclusion that the problem of defaulting was 'not so serious as the statistics [made] it appear'. Although it remained an 'important factor' in the spread of VD, the Committee was convinced by statistical evidence that most patients who discontinued treatment prematurely were no longer infectious.[43]

However, there was an increasing willingness within the medical profession to experiment with compulsory measures to secure treatment of VD.[44] Even the Trevethin Committee recommended that local health authorities might be permitted to experiment with 'special measures' for limited periods.[45] The question of compulsory measures was also raised in Parliament on several occasions.[46] In 1937, under continuing pressure from local authorities to introduce compulsory notification, the Ministry of Health sent an official commission to Denmark, Sweden and Norway (which employed compulsory treatment), and to Holland (which, like Britain, relied on a voluntary system), to investigate their VD policies. In their report, the commissioners, Colonel L.W. Harrison and D.C.L. Ward, both from the Ministry of Health, T. Ferguson from the Department of Health for Scotland, and Margaret Rorke, a VD consultant at the Royal Free Hospital London, reported that neither compulsory notification nor compulsory treatment were resisted in the Scandinavian countries. On the other hand, however, they concluded that compulsory treatment was not 'a major factor influencing the results of the anti-venereal measures in the countries where it [was] employed'.[47]

Consequently, as a first reaction of the Ministry of Health to the outbreak of the Second World War, a voluntarist strategy was maintained. VD treatment facilities were expanded and a new education campaign was launched.[48] At the beginning of 1940, the Ministry of Health firmly rejected any regulations for following up defaulters or tracing contacts of infected persons on the grounds that this would endanger the doctor–patient relation.[49] It was only in November 1942 that, under Defence of the Realm Act (DORA), Regulation 33B, the British Government finally adopted an emergency measure designed to notify named contacts of infected patients and to penalise such contacts who refused to submit to examination and treatment.[50] Thereby, the Ministry of Health hoped to bring under medical treatment those 'who [had] shown themselves unresponsive to educational work or to methods of persuasion and who, owing to this refusal to undertake treatment, remain[ed] a constant source of danger to the health of the community' and a threat to military power in war time.[51] Compulsory notification of VD, although repeatedly demanded by local authorities in 1943, was not introduced. As explained by the Minister of Health, Ernest Brown, this was, first, because of 'a long tradition of secrecy and silence' in Britain, secondly because of the danger 'that patients would be reluctant to seek proper medical advice', and thirdly because some doctors would be reluctant to notify because of the 'moral implication of the diseases'.[52] In practice, only a relatively small number of people, mainly women, were affected by DORA 33B. In 1944, 8,339 contacts (of whom only 246 were men) were reported under the regulation. However, only 82 people were prosecuted for refusing medical examination or for discontinuing treatment prematurely.[53] Nevertheless, DORA 33B unleashed again protest from women's, social purity, and Church organisations and was subsequently revoked in December 1947.[54] Cabinet sub-committees also reviewed the issue of broader controls with which to discipline defaulters and venereal recidivists in 1943 and 1944,[55] largely in response to Scottish health pressure groups. But yet again, the outcome of VD politics in England and Wales from the Second World War onwards was a commitment to voluntarism, and a fundamental reliance on the traditional voluntary strategies of treatment and health education, supplemented by voluntary contact tracing.

## Scotland

A S IN ENGLAND, the basis of VD policy in twentieth-century Scotland was the Public Health VD regulations of 1916 which required local authorities to provide free, voluntary and confidential diagnosis and treatment at VD clinics.[56] They were also required to educate the public in the causes and effects of VD and in the means of prevention. No legal compulsion was involved, and Scottish VD and STD measures have never been underpinned by specific powers of compulsion. Although, under Scottish Law, the deliberate communication of any infectious disease is indictable as an assault, apart from a brief period in 1918 under DORA 40D, no legislation existed to penalise its accidental transmission. VD remained outside the statutory definition of notifiable diseases. A person venereally infected was not legally obliged to seek or sustain treatment, nor to disclose his/her sexual contacts. Moreover, even when such contacts were traced, apart from a short period from 1942–47 when, as in England, DORA 33B operated, there was no power to compel them to submit to examination and treatment.

Nevertheless, one of the more distinctive features of twentieth-century Scottish medical history has been the strong compulsionist tradition surrounding the discussion and administration of VD. From the 1920s, a succession of campaigns in Scotland was fought by health authorities and civic leaders for legal powers to combat the spread of VD. In the 1920s, three separate bills were advanced seeking to notify, detain and penalise infected persons, and the parents of infected children, who refused to seek medical advice or to sustain a course of treatment until certified as non-infective.[57] These were proposals that were resisted and frustrated by the English Ministry of Health in Whitehall and Westminster. Subsequently, a fresh campaign was launched during the Second World War, culminating in heated confrontation between the Scottish Office and Ministry of Health in the War Cabinet.[58] As late as 1968, Scottish politicians and civic leaders were still pressing for the law to play a more proactive role in the containment of VD.

Perhaps more significantly, at the level of the local State, moral panic surrounding VD in Scotland provided the peg upon which to hang a range of bye-laws and administrative procedures regulating patterns of social intercourse well into the second half of the twentieth century. In the Scottish cities, public order, public morality and public health remained inextricably linked both administratively and ideologically, and this shaped a wide-ranging local statutory framework regulating a range of social spaces and behaviours that offended the precepts of social hygiene. Thus, VD was central to the formulation of regulations not only with respect to prostitution and soliciting, but also on the layout and conduct of places of refreshment and entertainment such as ice-cream parlours and dance halls, and the moral hygiene of lodging houses.[59]

The use of the law was highly discriminatory and was targeted at the young, and predominantly at so-called working-class 'problem' girls and promiscuous women. For example, in inter-war Scotland, local welfare and police authorities commonly interpreted the Mental Deficiency Act of 1913 so as to institutionalise girls who became pregnant or contracted VD as 'moral imbeciles' who threatened racial degeneration. Similarly, powers of medical inspection under the Criminal Justice Act of 1948, introduced as an aid to sentencing, were later exploited to ensure that girls and young women charged with soliciting were regularly medically examined for VD by public health doctors. Likewise, until the late 1960s, the Children and Young Persons Act was used to refer to VD clinics as a matter of routine all girls committed to remand homes and approved schools, irrespective of whether they were displaying any symptoms.[60]

A range of explanations might be advanced to explain this very close association between VD policy and the law in Scotland. It was not primarily a function of the incidence of VD as, until the 1980s, the incidence of VD and STDs in Scotland was, if anything, lower than in England and Wales. A more probable explanation may lie in long-standing social and institutional attitudes to sexuality and venereal infection and a strong tradition of civic authoritarianism and interventionism in Scotland. As early as 1497, repressive controls were introduced by Aberdeen Town Council and the Privy Council of Scotland to contain the spread of syphilis or 'grandgore', as it was commonly called. As in most subsequent regulations, the Aberdeen edict especially targeted sexually active women, demanding that 'all loose women disist from their vices and syn of venerie' on pain of being branded or being banished from the town. Subsequently, this commitment to the regulation and containment of pestilential infections was sustained by the Scottish Royal Burghs and further consolidated by Scottish local government authorities in the nineteenth century. Scottish medical and legal ideology had been heavily influenced by the European enlightenment, and the German tradition of 'medical police' clearly influenced Scottish health administration.[61] Medical Officers of Health were primarily appointed to aid the police and the magistracy, and this ideological and institutional conflation of public health and moral order was to prove decisive in defining the response of the central and local State to the threat of VD in modern Scotland.

Twentieth-century procedures also drew on a long tradition of penalising the transmission of VD under Scottish Common Law. In Scottish Civil Law, the communication of VD by a husband to his wife was held to entitle the wife to separation on the grounds of cruelty.[62] In addition, under Scottish Criminal Law, the communication of VD was treated as an aggravation of sexual offences such as rape and libidinous practices involving young girls.[63] The belief in ridding oneself of disease by means of transference was embedded in Scottish folk medicine and none more so than the widespread and enduring belief that VD could be cured by intercourse with a virgin.[64] As a result, the early twentieth-century legal system in

Scotland continued to view VD as much as a facet of criminal assault as a threat to social hygiene.

Underlying this more legalistic stance of Scottish health and welfare authorities was also a powerful moral agenda drawing in part upon a vigorous tradition of church and community disciplining of sexual behaviour. Former patterns of church discipline administered by the kirk sessions and most vividly reflected in the stool of penitence had been largely undermined by 1900, but their spirit lived on well into the twentieth century. Indeed, the views of the Churches, and especially of what was depicted as an 'illiberal presbyterian theocracy', remained highly influential in the formulation of socio-moral policy in Scotland well after the Second World War.[65] Although the United Free Church feared that VD controls might lead to the concealment of disease and that the legal process might obscure more fundamental issues of personal morality, the Church of Scotland strongly endorsed the campaign for compulsion. In the view of its Church and Nation Committee, while the 'clear, reverent teaching of the true function of sex in human life and the intimate and sacred relationship between body and spirit was vital', there was also an urgent need to protect the family and the community against defaulters and libertines.[66] This contrasted with the voluntarist stance traditionally adopted by leaders of the Church of England.

The ideology and social leverage of medical expertise within Scottish society was also a factor. The ideology of professional expertise shaping the Social Hygiene Movement in Scotland was, as in other countries with compulsionist leanings, such as Germany and France, heavily influenced by Eugenics and its more coercive prescriptions for the 'degenerate'.[67] It envisaged an interventionist role by medicine and the law whereby nurse almoners and social work agencies would work in liaison with the clinics, and with the courts and the police, to identify and monitor key vectors of the disease. As in Germany, Scottish public health officials and venereologists often brought to the problem of VD an aggressive professional imperialism in their campaign to eradicate racial poisons, and often saw the law as an essential backstop to deal with venereal recidivists and 'problem girls' who appeared immune to the normal processes of treatment and VD propaganda.[68] Thus, for Dr David Lees, Clinical Medical Officer in charge of Edinburgh's VD Scheme, and the most influential Scottish venereologist of the inter-war period, 'what was needed was not a discontinuance of the voluntary system, but a strengthening of it; not an infringement of the liberty of any subject who deserved liberty, but definitely and avowedly an infringement of the liberty of the libertine'.[69] Such views were typical of a generation of social hygienists operating in the field of public health, whose outlook towards VD had been shaped by service in the medical corps during the First World War, and who were concerned to establish the professional status of their expertise.

Moreover, in contrast to the English experience, many strands of the Women's Movement in Scotland were sympathetic to VD controls. This may have had something to do with the fact that, although local police acts, such as the Glasgow Police Act of 1866, had been widely used to coerce prostitutes,[70] the Contagious Diseases Acts had not applied in nineteenth-century Scotland and thus the anti-regulationist tradition was weaker. Certainly, Scottish branches of many women's organisations, such as the Women's Citizens Association and National Council of Women, were more receptive to measures that might protect the welfare of women and children from the negligent spread of VD and were less hostile to the efforts of magistrates and clinicians to restrain sexual delinquents and defaulters.[71]

Above all, it was the relative autonomy of the Scottish cities well into the twentieth century that enabled this culture of interventionism to feed through into bye-laws and local bills in which VD as a health issue was regularly mobilised in the policing of public morality. Early twentieth-century commentators compared Edinburgh and Glasgow to the city states of classical antiquity, and along with Aberdeen and Dundee, they continued to shape public health and public order policy to a far greater degree than their English and Welsh counterparts. Moreover, they fought to preserve this autonomy as part of a continuing battle to secure a Scottish identity in health affairs, and the pursuit of a self-consciously distinct, compulsionist policy towards VD reflected that struggle. Thus, the campaign for compulsory notification and treatment in the 1920s was a conscious revolt against what was perceived to be the libertarian fears and moral laxity of 'the cathedral cities south of the border' and the vacillating voluntarism of an English Ministry of Health. And this distinctively interventionist ideology towards VD became a constant reference point for Scottish nationalists from the 1920s through until the 1960s in their battles to obtain freedom from Whitehall and Westminster.[72] Interestingly, this association between a more interventionist and legalistic stance towards sexual health and social hygiene and the quest for regional or national identity was paralleled in other countries such as New Zealand and Australia, and notably in Weimar Germany.[73]

## Conclusion

HOPEFULLY, THIS BRIEF EXAMINATION of the forces shaping VD policy has teased out some of the key variables in determining the relationship in any one country between the law, medicine and sexual morality and its relative weighting of public health priorities and civil liberties. In this paper, we have posited a range of positions, with Germany at one compulsionist extreme and England at the libertarian end of the spectrum, with Scotland located somewhere in between. Clearly, at one level, the contrast between the more coercive strategy adopted towards VD in Germany and the more voluntarist approach in England can be explained with reference to political traditions. Germany had a long tradition of State intervention in public health policy whereas in England it encountered strong resistance from libertarian forces.[74] In particular, the history of the Contagious Diseases Acts continued to haunt English policy makers and to constrain interventionist initiatives.

However, a rather aggregative and simplistic picture has, of necessity, been given. A more detailed analysis would indicate more clearly the continuing divisions in all these countries over the issue of VD controls, especially within professional opinion. Thus, as has been seen, in Germany even after 1927, there were strands of professional and public opinion that remained sceptical of the value of compulsion and concerned over the issue of confidentiality. Conversely, in England, there was always a vocal minority of clinicians and Medical Officers of Health advocating more stringent measures to control what they perceived to be the key vectors of the diseases. Indeed, certain health authorities, such as those in Bradford and Liverpool, produced very similar proposals to those advanced in Scotland. Moreover, in many countries at both ends of the compulsionist-voluntarist spectrum, there was significant concern over the role and power of the expert in society and a reluctance to arm medical science and officialdom with powers of legal coercion. Significantly, such reservations were often most vehemently expressed by lawyers themselves who, then as now in the case of HIV and AIDS, could readily appreciate the legal hazards of imposing controls in an area of medicine in which the technologies of diagnosis, treatment, and cure remained contentious, and in which confidentiality remained the linchpin of patient rights and compliance.[75]

# Notes

1   Studies of this process include, L. Bland, '"Cleansing the Portals of Life": The Venereal Disease Campaign in the early Twentieth Century' in M. Langan and B. Schwarz (eds.), *Crises in the British State, 1880–1930* (London, 1985), ch. 9; A. Brandt, *No Magic Bullet, A Social History of Venereal Disease in the United States since 1880* (Oxford, 1985); R.C. Bolea, 'Venereal Diseases in Spain during the last third of the Nineteenth Century: An Approach to the Moral Bases of Public Health', *Dynamis*, 11 (1991) 239–62; A. Corbin, *Women for Hire: Prostitution and Sexuality in France after 1850* (Cambridge, MA and London, 1990), ch. 6; P.J. Fleming, 'Fighting the "Red Plague": Observations on the Response to Venereal Disease in New Zealand 1910–45', *New Zealand Journal of History*, 22 (1988), 56–64; A. Mooij, *Out of Otherness: Characters and Narrators in the Dutch Venereal Disease Debates, 1850–1990* (Amsterdam and Atlanta, 1999), ch. 1; M. Murnane and K. Daniels, 'Prostitutes as "Purveyors of Disease": Venereal Disease Legislation in Tasmania 1868–1945', *Hecate*, 5 (1979), 5–21; C. Quétel, *History of Syphilis* (Cambridge, 1990) chs. 6–7; L. Sauerteig, *Krankeit, Sexualität, Gesellschaft: Geschlechtskrankheiten und Gesundheitspolitik in Deutschland im 19. frühen 20. Jahrhundert* (Stuttgart, 1999); M. Spongberg, *Feminizing Venereal Disease: The Body of the Prostitute in Nineteenth-Century Medical Discourse* (London, 1997); P. Weindling, *Health, Race and German Politics Between National Unification and Nazism, 1870–1945* (Cambridge, 1989), ch. 3. Roger Davidson is indebted to the Wellcome Trust, and Lutz Sauerteig to the German Historical Institute, London, and the German Academic Exchange Service, whose financial assistance made possible much of the research upon which this paper is based.

2   For an historical overview, see G.S. Meyer, 'Criminal Punishment for the Transmission of Sexually Transmitted Diseases: Lessons from Syphilis', *Bulletin of the History of Medicine and Allied Sciences*, 65 (1991), 549–64.

3   On methodological aspects of comparative research, see L. Sauerteig, 'Vergleich: Ein Königsweg auch für die Medizingeschichte? Methodologische Fragen vergleichenden Forschens' in N. Paul and T. Schlich (eds.), *Medizingeschichte: Aufgaben, Probleme, Perspektiven* (Frankfurt/M and New York, 1998).

4   See on Germany, Sauerteig, *Krankheit, Sexualität, Gesellschaft*, pp. 318–42; on England, 'Editorial' in *Health & Empire*, 1, No. 3 (January/February 1922), 18; J.F. Blackett, 'The Case for the Notification of Venereal Disease', *Medical Officer*, 30 (1923), 193–94.

5   'Regulativ über die sanitätspolizeilichen Vorschriften der am häufigsten vorkommenden Krankheiten', 8 April 1835, paragraph 65, in F.L. Augustin, *Die Königlich preussische Medicinialverfassung, oder vollständige Darstellung aller, das Medicinalwesen und die medcinische Polizei in den Königlich Preussischen Staaten betreffenden Gesetze, Verordnungen und Einrichtungen*, Vol. 4 (Potsdam & Berlin, 1838), pp. 978–80. See Alfred Blaschko, 'Hygiene der Geschlechtskrankheiten' in A. Gärtner (ed.), *Weyls Handbuch der Hygiene*, Vol. 8 (Leipzig, 2nd edition

1918–22), pp. 415–16; A. Fischer, *Geschichte des deutschen Gesundheitswesens*, Vol. 2 (Berlin, 1933), pp. 562, 578.

6   See R.J. Evans, *Death in Hamburg: Society and Politics in the Cholera-Years 1830–1910* (Oxford, 1987).

7   'Gesetz zur Bekämpfung der gemeingefährlichen Krankheiten', 30 June 1900, *Reichsgesetzblatt* (1900).

8   See, for example, the joint petition of the Berlin and Hamburg Branch of the International Abolitionist Federation and the Verein Frauenwohl, April 1900, Bundesarchiv Berlin (BAB), 15.01/11900, p. 39. On the German abolitionists, see L. Sauerteig, 'Frauenemanzipation und Sittlichkeit. Die Rezeption des englischen Abolitionismus in Deutschland' in R. Muhs, J. Paulmann and W. Steinmetz (eds.), *Aneignung und Abwehr. Interkultureller Transfer zwischen Deutschland und Grossbritannien im 19. Jahrhundert* (Bodenheim, 1998).

9   Motion of the Centre Party to amend paragraph 327a of the Imperial Penal Law, *Stenographische Berichte über die Verhandlungen des Deutschen Reichstags* (VDtRT), Vol. 172, No. 31, p. 180. See Sauerteig, *Krankheit, Sexualität, Gesellschaft*, pp. 360–67.

10  F.v. Liszt, 'Der strafrechtliche Schutz gegen Gesundheitsgefährdung durch Geschlechtskranke Gutachten', *Zeitschrift für Bekämpfung der Geschlechtskrankheiten*, 1 (1903), pp. 1–25; A. Neisser, *Die Geschlechtskrankheiten und ihre Bekämpfung. Vorschläge und Forderungen für Ärzte und Soziologen* (Berlin, 1916), pp. 128–30.

11  The *Königliches Landgericht* in Munich sentenced a man to five months imprisonment in 1903 because he infected a girl with syphilis and gonorrhoea. *Sammlung gerichtlicher Entscheidungen auf dem Gebiete der öffentlichen Gesundheitspflege*, 5 (1908), 179.

12  'Verordnung zur Bekämpfung der Geschlechtskrankheiten', 11 December 1918, *Reichsgesetzblatt* (1918), No. 184, pp. 1431–32. A similar regulation was also included in the Imperial Act for Combatting VD of 1927.

13  Motion of Katharina Scheven in *Der Abolitionist*, 7 (1908), 11–16; R. Schmölder, 'Strafrechtliche und civilrechtliche Bedeutung der Geschlechtskrankheiten', *Zeitschrift für Bekämpfung der Geschlechtskrankheiten*, 1 (1903), pp. 73–94; Neisser, *Geschlechtskrankheiten*, pp. 128–30; 'Sachverständigenkommission der Deutschen Gesellschaft zur Bekämpfung der Geschlechtskrankheiten', *Zeitschrift für Bekämpfung der Geschlechtskrankheiten* (1916/17), pp. 100–27; meeting of the Imperial Health Council, 4 and 5 March 1908, BAB, 15.01/11866, pp. 232–54. On the history of the German Society for Combating VD, founded in 1902, see Sauerteig, *Krankheit, Sexualiät, Gesellschaft*, pp. 89–125.

14  Report of the 10th Parliamentary Committee on Population, VDtRT, Vol. 411, No. 2714, pp. 11–12; K. Pohlen, 'Kriminalstatistik betr. das RGBG', *Mitteilungen der Deutschen Gesellschaft zur Bekämpfung der Geschlechtskrankheiten*, 31 (1933), 88–96.

15 Report of the 16th Parliamentary Committee on Population, 7 July 1918, *VDtRT*, Vol. 321, No. 912, p. 1712; enactment of the Prussian War Ministry, 14 July 1915, and of the Bavarian War Ministry, 19 August 1915, Bayerisches Hauptstaatsarchiv, IV, MKr10103.

16 'Gesetz zur Bekämpfung der Geschlechtskrankheiten', 22 February 1927, *Reichsgesetzblatt* (1927), part I, No. 9. For extracts from the Act, see H. Haustein, 'The German Federal Law for Combatting Venereal Diseases', *Health & Empire*, New Series 2 (1927), 89–99.

17 See 'Gesetz zur Bekämpfung der Geschlechtskrankheiten', 23 July 1953, *Bundesgesetzblatt* (1953), part I, p. 700.

18 365th meeting, 14 June 1923, *VDtRT*, Vol. 360, col. 11354.

19 See Sauerteig, *Krankheit, Sexualität, Gesellschaft*, ch. IV.3.

20 F.B. Smith, 'The Contagious Diseases Acts Reconsidered', *Social History of Medicine*, 3 (1990), 197–215; J.R. Walkowitz, *Prostitution and Victorian Society. Women, Class, and the State* (Cambridge, 1980); P. McHugh, *Prostitution and Victorian Social Reform* (New York, 1980).

21 Sauerteig, *Krankheit, Sexualität, Gesellschaft*, pp. 379–419.

22 R.W. Johnstone, *Report on Venereal Diseases, Parliamentary Papers, 1913* (Cd.7029) *XXXII*, pp. 27–28.

23 Arthur Newsholme, in his introduction to Johnstone, *Report*, p. iv. On Newsholme and his views on VD, see J.M. Eyler, *Sir Arthur Newsholme and State Medicine, 1885–1935* (Cambridge, 1997), pp. 277–94.

24 *Final Report of the Royal Commission on Venereal Diseases, P.P. 1916* (Cd. 8189) *XVI*, pp. 50, 65. See also R.R. Willcox, 'Fifty Years Since the Conception of an Organized Venereal Diseases Service in Great Britain. The Royal Commission of 1916', *British Journal of Venereal Disease*, 43 (1967), 1–9.

25 The Public Health (Venereal Diseases) Regulation, 1916, 12 July 1916, *Statutory Rules and Orders* (1916), Vol. 3, pp. 74–76; Local Government Board, *Venereal Diseases Circulars*, 13 July 1916 (London, 1916); Public Record Office (PRO), MH55/531, MH55/532. On the background, see Eyler, *Arthur Newsholme*, pp. 277–78, 284–90.

26 PRO, MH55/185; *Sixth Annual Report of the Ministry of Health, P.P. 1924–25* (Cmd.2724) *XI*, pp. 7, 143, *Eleventh Annual Report of the Ministry of Health, P.P. 1930–31* (Cmd.3667) *XIII*, pp. 58, 236. D. Evans, 'Tackling the "Hideous Scourge": The Creation of the Venereal Disease Treatment Centres in Early Twentieth-Century Britain', *Social History of Medicine* 5 (1992), 413–33.

27 L. Sauerteig, 'Moralismus versus Pragmatismus: Die Kontroverse um Schutzmittel gegen Geschlechtskrankheiten zu Beginn des 20. Jahrhunderts im deutsch-englischen Vergleich' in M. Dinges and T. Schlich (eds.), *Neue Wege in der Seuchengeschichte* (Stuttgart, 1995), pp. 207–47; B.A. Towers, 'Health Education

Policy 1916–1926: Venereal Disease and the Prophylaxis Dilemma', *Medical History*, 24 (1980), 70–87.

28 *Final Report of the Royal Commission*, p. 50.

29 PRO, CAB 23/5WC52(18)10, p. 122, 22 February 1918; PRO, CAB M8/23/ 5WC365(18)14, p. 159, 13 March 1918; Debate in the House of Commons on the Criminal Law Amendment Bill, *Hansard*, *[HC]* 90, 19 February 1917, cols. 1098–131; Association for Moral and Social Hygiene, Fawcett Library, London Guildhall University, AMSH 311/2. See also L. Sauerteig, 'Sex, Medicine and Morality during the First World War' in M. Harrison and R. Cooter (eds.), *War, Medicine and Modernity, 1860–1945* (Stroud, 1998); Bland, *Cleansing the Portals of Life*, pp. 203–4; S. Buckley, 'The Failure to Resolve the Problem of Venereal Disease Among the Troops in Britain During World War I' in B. Bond and I. Roy (eds.), *War and Society. A Yearbook of Military History*, Vol. 2 (London, 1977), pp. 65–85; E.H. Beardsley, 'Allied Against Sin. American and British Responses to Venereal Disease in World War I', *Medical History*, 20 (1976), 189–202.

30 H.W. Bayly, *Venereal Disease: Its Prevention, Symptoms and Treatment* (London, 1920), pp. 1–4; E.T. Burke (VD Officer to the County Borough of Warrington), *The Venereal Problem* (London, 1919), ch. 14; *The Medical Officer*, 24 (1920), 46; 26 (1922), 78, 173; Blackett (Medical Officer of Health, Bath), *Notification of Venereal Disease*. On the Society for the Prevention of VD, founded in October 1919, and its quarrel with the NCCVD about prophylaxis, see Sauerteig, *Moralismus versus Pragmatismus*, pp. 225–32.

31 O. May, *The Prevention of Venereal Disease* (Oxford, 1918), pp. 154–57.

32 NCCVD Executive Committee, Minutes, 23 June 1920, Contemporary Medical Archive Centre (CMAC), Wellcome Institute for the History of Medicine, SA/BSH/A 2/4.

33 *Health & Empire*, 1, No. 3 (January/February 1922); No. 6 (May 1922), 47–50 with several papers pro (mainly from physicians and Medical Officers of Health in larger cities) and contra (from members of social purity organisations and Medical Officers of Health in rural areas) presented at a VD Conference organised by the City of London Corporation.

34 Sauerteig, *Moralismus versus Pragmatismus*, pp. 224–32.

35 For example, BSHC Executive Committee Minutes, 4 July 1927, 6 February 1928, CMAC, SA/BSH/A2/10; PRO, MH55/1326, note of a meeting in the Ministry of Health with BSHC delegation, 4 June 1937.

36 C.J. Bond, 'The Attitude of the State and Society to Anti-Social Diseases', *Health & Empire*, 1, New Series (1926), 47–48.

37 E.T. Burke, 'Are we to have Compulsory Treatment of Venereal Disease?', *Health & Empire*, New Series 10 (1935),120–23.

38 BSHC Executive Committee, Minutes, 1 February 1932, CMAC, SA/BSH/A2/13.

39 'A Threat of Compulsion!', *Health & Empire*, New Series, 12 (1937), 1.

40  B. Blackett, 'Progress in Social Hygiene 1914–35', *Health & Empire*, New Series, 10 (1935), 179.

41  'A Threat of Compulsion!', 2.

42  See, for example, the statement of the Chief Medical Officer in the Ministry of Health, George Newman, 'The Present Position of Government Action in Venereal Disease' in *Proceedings of the Imperial Social Hygiene Congress at the British Empire Exhibition, May 12th–16th, 1924* (London, 1924), pp. 19–21.

43  *Report of the Committee of Inquiry on Venereal Disease* (London, 1923), pp. 7–8. See Towers, 'Health Education Policy', 83–84.

44  See, for example, *Health & Empire*, New Series, 3 (1928), 173–74; R. Forgan (Executive Medical Officer, Lanarkshire), 'Compulsory Treatment of Venereal Diseases', *Medical Officer*, 39 (1928), 269–71.

45  *Report of the Committee of Inquiry*, p. 10. The controversial Edinburgh Corporation Bill of 1928 was viewed by many observers as consistent with such a recommendation.

46  See *Hansard*, [HC] 301, 2 May 1935, cols. 537–38; 7 May 1935, col. 817; 324 , 8 June 1937, cols. 1661, 1670, 1713–14; 325, 17 June 1937, col. 549.

47  L.W. Harrison, D.C.L. Ward, T. Ferguson, Margaret Rorke, *Report on Anti-Venereal Measures in Certain Scandinavian Countries and Holland* (London, 1938), p. 120.

48  See PRO MH55/1384, 1333, 1334; Ministry of Health, 'Circular No 1956', 26 January 1940, in *Medical Officer*, 63 (1940), 42–43; D. Shields, 'War Conditions and Venereal Disease: The Recent Ministry Circular', ibid., 159–60; Fawcett Library, AMSH 310/1, Ministry of Health, 'Circular No 2727', 8 January 1943.

49  See PRO, MH55/1385.

50  Emergency Powers (Defence) General Regulations, 5 November 1942, *Statutory Rules and Orders* (1942), Vol. 2, pp. 89–94. On the discussion over DORA 33B see PRO, MH55/1326.

51  Ministry of Health to Medical Officers of Health, 'Compulsory Treatment of Venereal Disease', 8 January 1943, Fawcett Library, AMSH 310/1.

52  Ernest Brown to T. Harry Hewlett, 4 January 1943, PRO, MH55/1326.

53  L.W. Harrison, 'Venereal Diseases' in A.S. MacNalty (ed.), *The Civilian Health and Medical Services*, Vol. 1 (London, 1953), pp. 120–21.

54  PRO, MH55/1347 and MH55/1350; Fawcett Library, AMSH 310/1 and 310/2; Association for Moral and Social Hygiene (ed.), *Regulation 33B. The Medical Aspect, the Legal Aspect, the Social Aspect* (London, 1943).

55  Harrison, *Venereal Diseases*, pp. 121–22.

56  *Local Government Board for Scotland, Venereal Diseases Circulars*, 31 October 1916 (Edinburgh, 1916).

57 For a detailed discussion of these proposals, see R. Davidson, '"A Scourge to be firmly gripped": The Campaign for VD Controls in Interwar Scotland', *Social History of Medicine*, 6 (1993), 213–35.

58 R. Davidson, 'Fighting "the Deadly Scourge": The Impact of World War II on Civilian VD policy in Scotland', *Scottish Historical Review*, 75 (1996), 72–97.

59 See, for example, *Public General Acts, 1 and 2 Geo.5, Ch. 51, Burgh Police (Scotland) Amendment Act, 1911; Local and Private Acts, 3&4 Geo.5, Ch. LXXIV, Edinburgh Corporation Act, 1913*.

60 R. Davidson, 'Venereal Disease, Sexual Morality, and Public Health in Interwar Scotland', *Journal of the History of Sexuality*, 5 (1994) 267–94; D.H.H. Robertson and G. George, 'Medical and Legal Problems in the Treatment of Delinquent Girls in Scotland', *British Journal of Venereal Diseases*, 46 (1970), 46–51.

61 B. White, 'Training Medical Policemen: Forensic Medicine and Public Health in Nineteenth-Century Scotland' in M. Clark and C. Crawford (eds.), *Legal Medicine in History* (Cambridge, 1994), pp.145–63.

62 P. Fraser, *Treatise on Husband and Wife According to the Law of Scotland, Vol.2*, 2nd edition (Edinburgh, 1878), p. 891.

63 J. Chisholm (ed.), *Green's Encyclopaedia of the Law of Scotland* (Edinburgh, 1911), p. 492.

64 Giving evidence to the Glasgow High Court in 1913, Dr James Devon, Prison Surgeon, claimed to have discovered the belief 'among people of different places and occupations – so different that now [he would] scarcely be surprised to come across it anywhere'.

65 K.M. Boyd, *Scottish Church Attitudes to Sex, Marriage and the Family* (Edinburgh, 1980), pp. 4–12; C.G. Brown, *The People in the Pews: Religion and Society in Scotland since 1780* (Dundee, 1993), pp. 44–45.

66 Church of Scotland, *Reports to General Assembly* (1944), pp. 280–81.

67 P. Weindling, 'Sexually Transmitted Diseases between Imperial and Nazi Germany', *Genitourinary Medicine*, 70 (1994) 284–85; Corbin, *Women for Hire*, ch. 6.

68 Davidson, 'A Scourge to be Firmly Gripped', 216–18; Davidson, 'Venereal Disease, Sexual Morality and Public Health', 280–82.

69 *British Medical Journal*, II (1928), 64–65.

70 L. Mahood, *The Magdalenes: Prostitution in the Nineteenth Century* (London & New York, 1990), ch, 7.

71 Davidson, 'A Scourge to be Firmly Gripped', 221–22.

72 See, for example, Scottish Record Office, HH65/122/60, Evidence of Scottish Covenant Association to Royal Commission on Scottish Affairs, 22 October 1953.

73 P.J. Fleming, 'Fighting the "Red Plague": Observations on the Response to Venereal Disease in New Zealand 1910–45', *New Zealand Journal of History*, 22 (1988), 60; D.R. Tibbits, *The Medical, Social and Political Response to Venereal Diseases in Victoria*

*1860–1980* (Ph.D. dissertation, Monash University, 1994), p. 161; Weindling, *Health, Race and German Politics*, p. 289.

74  C. Hamlin, 'State Medicine in Great Britain' in D. Porter (ed.), *The History of Public Health and the Modern State* (Amsterdam, 1994), pp. 132–64; R.M. Macleod. 'Law, Medicine and Public Opinion: The Resistance to Compulsory Health Legislation 1870–1907', *Public Law* (1967), 107–28, 189–211.

75  R. Porter and D. Porter, 'AIDS: Law, Liberty and Public Health' in P. Byrne (ed.), *Health, Rights and Resources* (London, 1988), 76–93; R. Bayer and L. Gostin, 'Legal and Ethical Issues in AIDS' in M.S. Gottlieb et al., *Current Topics in AIDS, Volume 2* (Chichester, 1989), pp. 263–83.

# Defining Brain Death:
# The German Debate
# in Historical Perspective

*Claudia Wiesemann*

'CANNIBALS AT THE CADAVER?'[1] 'Do transplantation surgeons gut human bodies that are still alive?'[2] Recently German readers have become more and more familiar with headlines like these. Television and the print media attack scientists for trespassing natural and moral limits and imposing risks on society that cannot be controlled rationally. Astonishingly, the concept of brain death is heavily disputed in Germany nowadays although it was introduced into clinical practice nearly thirty years ago and has been used ever since without significant public objections.

Since 1968 a person has been called brain dead whose brain is completely and irreversibly damaged. Brain death was regarded as the essential criterion for the death of a human being. It was meant to replace former criteria of death such as the arrest of cardiac and pulmonary functions. It had been established to obviate artificial respiration in hopeless cases and to facilitate organ procurement for transplantation. An understanding of the use of the concept of brain death by scientists, lawyers, and the public during the last three decades may help to shed light on the social role of science in modern and late-modern societies. How was it treated by medical scientists in the late sixties when heart transplantation led to an urgent need for a new definition of death? How was it accepted by the public, introduced into clinical routine, and implemented through medical and legal policies? And why was this public consensus definitely questioned in the last four or five years? This paper does not focus on the scientific meaning of the concept of brain death. Instead, it will be treated as a social phenomenon, as the pivot for a radical shift in power between doctors and patients. By establishing brain death as the essential criterion for the death of a human being, the determination of death became a question of solely medical expertise, something that could be exerted and controlled only by medical experts. Whereas death in the traditional manner by cardiac or respiratory arrest could be identified by any sensible person, the diagnosis of brain death could only be made by specially skilled physicians. Moreover, the explantation of organs substantially increased the importance of this shift in competency. Normally the dead body was laid out for some days before the funeral. Anybody could satisfy himself about the physical reality of death and also the possibility of recovery from suspended animation. After the removal of organs from a brain dead person, however, nobody could falsify the doctors' judgement. People's attitude towards this change in social competency is affected by their attitude towards medical science and the role of science in society. To explain this in detail, reference will be made to Ulrich Beck's social theory of simple and reflexive modernisation. Beck described his theory of late modern social attitudes towards science in *Risikogesellschaft* (1986), *Die Erfindung des Politischen* (1993) and *Reflexive Modernization*.[3]

According to Beck the social structures of today can be characterised by the management of risks. Risk society is a product of the ongoing process of modernisation, but its characteristics are completely different from those of simple modernity, although it has evolved from simple modernity not by revolution but 'by virtue of its inherent dynamism'.[4] Simple modernity was the essential basis of the industrial society. It is characterised by the disembedding of tradition, the predominance of instrumental rationality, a linear model of progress and a belief in the rational control of the process of modernisation. Science and technology occupied the leading role in this development. Simple modernisation relied on a strict dichotomy between scientists and non-scientists, modernity and tradition, rationality and irrationality, and it was driven by the belief that problems occurring could be resolved by further scientific research. But previously unforeseen risks and the side effects of scientific progress gradually tended to undermine the idea of instrumental and rational control. The consequence of autonomous modernisation is a new type of uncertainty about the management of risks and the rationality of progress itself. This, according to Beck, is the beginning of reflexive modernity, 'a *radicalization* of modernity, which breaks up the premises and contours of industrial society and opens path to another modernity'[5]. Whereas in simple modernity scientific problems were objectified and rationalized as an incentive to more scientific research, in reflexive modernity the management of risks helps to demystify and demonopolize science. As scientific hypotheses for risk management become more and more complex they are losing credibility. The public has to decide between different plausible or probable scientific claims. In this situation political groups make use of scientific expertise and counterexpertise to push their favourite practical and legal solutions. This also entails a new distribution of social power. In the following Beck's theory will be used to analyse social attitudes towards the concept of brain death, especially the relationship of medicine and law in the social setting of simple and reflexive modernity.

Before December 1967 the need for a new definition of death had been addressed occasionally by anaesthetists and forensic pathologists.[6] Due to the rapid diffusion of artificial respiration in the fifties and sixties, intensive care medicine was confronted with patients with incurable diseases and severe brain damage who were kept alive by mechanical ventilation. Besides, few transplantation centres had begun to transplant kidneys from the newly dead. These organs were procured from patients with cardiac or pulmonary arrest who had been 're-animated' after some minutes to prevent the removable organs from lethal destruction.[7] Both practices raised questions about the nature of death. Was it right to call somebody alive who had lost all his brain functions, just because his heart would not stop beating regularly? Was it, on the other hand, right to call somebody dead whose heart had stopped beating but whose body was again 're-animated' and even put on a heart and lung machine to keep his organs alive?[8]

On 3 December 1967, the surgeon Christiaan Barnard from the Grote Schuur Hospital in Capetown, South Africa, transplanted the beating heart of the 24-year-old Denise Darwall, a victim of a car accident, to the 55-year-old Louis Washkansky, suffering from progressive heart failure.[9] The next day, the news had spread all over the world. Heart surgery reacted as if Barnard had kicked off an avalanche. Only three days later, Dr Adrian Kantrowitz from the Maimonides Medical Center in New York performed the operation on a 17-days-old baby. His colleague Norman E. Shumway from the University of Stanford, California, followed him one month later.[10] The German press media reacted enthusiastically. A headline on the front page of the rather conservative popular newspaper *Die Welt* read: 'Surgeons: Big Success'.[11] The news magazine *Der Spiegel* reported that 'Professor Barnard, the wiry surgeon with the Kennedy smile (his hobby: water-skiing) had undertaken the hitherto boldest venture in the art of surgery'.[12] Only ten days after the first heart transplantation, the *Frankfurter Allgemeine Zeitung*, a newspaper for the learned and conservative, stated that the future of this new surgical technique seemed to be very encouraging.[13]

Barnard's pioneering deed engendered a worldwide discussion on the nature of human death. The heart became the symbol of modernisation. Was it the centre of life and emotion, and the essence of personality, or just one of hundreds of muscles in the human body? Heart transplantation seemed to give a simple answer to that question. The basic assumption of modernised society was that the heart was nothing but a mechanical pump, a small but effective muscle, a twitching lump of flesh.[14] In January 1968 the *Frankfurter Allgemeine* summarised that 'a beating heart – as we know now – does not say anything about the true condition of its bearer at the limits of life'.[15] *Die Welt* emphasised that physicians 'will have to tackle the necessity to determine more exactly the boundary between life and death and the time when one is allowed to explant a human being's organs for transplantation'.[16] Problems in finding a new definition of death seemed to be only of secondary importance and should be rationally resolved in time. Despite some critical voices that condemned heart transplantation as hubris and against human nature, Barnard became a media star who was invited to medical conferences, interviews and television shows all over the world. The death of his first transplant patient Washkansky after 18 days and the failure of both American heart transplantations did not diminish his fame. When Barnard returned to South Africa on New Year's Day 1968 to perform his second operation on the dentist Philip Blaiberg, he was so optimistic about his success that he informed the press the day before the transplantation.[17]

In Germany the discussion about heart transplantation and the medical and legal need for a new concept of death has to be considered against the background of the modernisation of society. Conservative and leftist newspapers and magazines agreed generally that scientific progress was intrinsically positive. Even after the death of the first transplant patient Louis Washkansky on 21 December, journalists confirmed that the first heart transplantation had been 'a necessary experiment'. *Die Welt* reminded its readers that medicine 'owes its progress to men who had not been discouraged by set backs'.[18] In an atmosphere where even conservative modernisers felt optimistic about the capabilities of scientific research, medical scientists themselves were able to express their doubts and to discuss problems of heart transplantation and the determination of death in public. Leading surgeons and neurologists demanded caution on these issues. Rudolf Kautzky, head of the department of neurosurgery at the University of Hamburg, publicly warned against uncritical scientific optimism: 'Whoever wants to define the death of a human being has to define the essence of a human being and it is at least controversial whether this can be achieved with scientific exactitude.'[19] The Düsseldorf neurologist Eberhard Bay complained that Barnard had not done everything possible for Denise Darwall, the donor of the heart for Washkansky.[20] In a CBS television interview even Barnard himself had touched the issue of brain death rather cautiously. He said: '[...] *it is my opinion* that death occurs *presumably* when the brain is dead'.[21]

German surgeons were reluctant to repeat the transplantation experiment. Rudolf Zenker, the president of the German Society of Surgery who was also head of one of the leading German transplantation teams in Munich and had pioneered kidney transplantation, appeared to be rather disinclined to transplant a heart.[22] The surgeon and Nobel prize winner Werner Forssmann condemned heart transplantation as an example of the decline in moral standards that was deemed to fail because of the unsolved immunological problems. Doctors would become slaughterers of their patients because the border between life and death could now easily be manipulated.[23] The leftist news magazine *Der Spiegel*, therefore, attacked both Zenker and Forssmann harshly for being old-fashioned and irrational. The news magazine denounced every critic of Barnard as a representative of 'a fatal tradition of mawkish idealism and irrationalism'[24] and complained that German surgeons 'who had formerly been quite progressive are now criticising Barnard from a moral point of view'.[25] It proved to be the most radical opinion leader in the process of modernisation. According to *Der Spiegel* the water-skiing Barnard, who was seen in discos, danced with Heidi Brühl, and had lunch with Gina Lollobrigida, represented the new type of thoroughly modern physician. Moreover, the news magazine reported approvingly that Barnard 'did not talk about ethos when he meant fees'.[26] At times when the political system in Germany was stirred by students' protests, the leftist magazine welcomed the opportunity to attack the medical profession and its strong hierarchical structures for being old-fashioned.[27] Ethical considerations that did not agree with instrumental rationality were interpreted as atavisms from pre-modern times.

Determined modernisers could also be found among the theologians. German Catholic and Protestant theologians mostly did not object to heart transplantation or a new definition of death. Rather, they supported the idea that defining death was a purely scientific task. In a public round table discussion at the Annual Meeting of the German Society for Neurosurgery in June 1968 the professor of Catholic moral theology, Franz Böckle, declared: 'I wish to bear witness to the thesis that brain death equals human death, although I cannot say anything about [the medical aspects of] brain death. You [i.e. the physicians] are the only ones competent to answer the question what brain death really means. [...] But if you say to me that for us this is something valid and imperative that can be proven in a scientifically adequate way, then I can say that I am willing to accept [that]'[28]. Böckle obviously expressed a kind of religious belief in science. He confessed his faith in the scientific world view. The Protestant theologian Helmut Thielecke would not object to the 'achievement of modern medicine' to 'vitally conserve' bodies for transplantation because to him this was just a question of biology, not of anthropology or theology.[29] Thielecke, who held a chair of systematic theology and social ethics at Hamburg University, was convinced that consciousness was an objective criterion to determine the meaning of human life. Every person who had irreversibly lost consciousness could be considered dead. Thielecke called them 'empty receptacles' and argued in favour of the vital conservation of their bodies for future transplantation needs.[30] The director of the Schleswig-Holstein Protestant Academy, R. Krapp, admonished his fellow ministers to leave behind 'Granddad's theology' and to forget 'pseudo-christian' arguments against brain death that did not meet objective medical criteria. He criticised Forssmann's position as an attempt to hinder medical progress by non-medical arguments.[31] Given the scientific facts, it was up to the theologians to tackle the resulting moral problems, for example, how to deal with the donor's proxies or how to distribute spare organs. Finally, senior lawyers declared that it was the legitimate task of medicine to define death and that, from a legal point of view, 'nobody could object to the conclusion of modern medicine that human life is derived from the higher functions of the brain'.[32] The federal Minister of Justice, Gustav Heinemann, a social democrat, said he would expect medicine to deliver exact criteria for the new definition of death.[33]

The result was a quite paradoxical situation: firstly, whereas medical scientists obviously did not feel at ease with giving a new definition of death on purely medical grounds and asked for help from other fields of knowledge, theologians and lawyers stressed that they were not competent and expressed their belief in the power of rational scientific explanations.[34] Secondly, although physicians were still seriously discussing the necessary criteria and technical methods to determine an irreversible loss of brain function[35] and were also still wondering whether certainty could ever be reached in this question[36], the idea that death equals brain death had already been widely accepted in public.[37] This basic agreement had been reached, in fact, by ignoring a very essential misunderstanding. Lawyers thought that determining death should be a matter of scientific certainty. Therefore, they were talking about scientific 'knowledge', the 'determination of death', insights into the 'nature of death' and the 'truth' of the scientific concept.[38] Physicians, however, when talking about brain death often used quite a different type of vocabulary. They were looking for a 'definition of death', they 'presumed' or 'postulated' death, and they tried to reach an 'agreement' over the definition of death.[39] This was obviously not the language of the exact sciences. Nobody really seemed interested in clarifying this Babylonic confusion.[40] Once in a while lawyers felt the need to admonish the doctors to keep to a more scientific idiom. In a round table discussion on the determination of death the professor of criminal law at Munich University Paul Bockelmann complained: 'Sometimes, gentlemen [...] I have got the impression from your comments that you do not take your brain death quite seriously. I have heard somebody say the person who is brain dead dies or must die. I, however, think that the brain dead does not die or have to die, but the brain dead is dead – provided that the brain dead is dead by definition.'[41]

Indeed, physicians were not primarily aiming at scientific certitude but at a convincing practical solution. The first official statement on brain death by a commission of the German Society of Surgery was published in May 1968.[42] The statement fixed criteria for the diagnosis of brain death such as the irreversible loss of consciousness and of spontaneous respiration, and a flat EEG. The members of the commission intended to establish brain death as the binding criterion of death in every case, not just in case of irreversible coma and artificial respiration. They wished to replace completely the former heart-and-lung criteria by the new brain death criterion. Therefore, they declared that brain death could also 'be postulated' when patients with incurable diseases (but not necessarily with cerebral dysfunction) suffered a fatal heart attack. This was meant to avoid problems with explanting organs from non-heart-beating cadavers. If in such a case somebody was called dead because of his 'postulated' brain death, his heart and lung functions could be 're-animated' for organ procurement without blurring the nature of death.[43]

By the end of 1968, about one hundred heart transplantations had been performed already in different countries of the world such as the United States, France, Brazil or Spain, forty of them in the last two months.[44] But the long-term results were not at all encouraging. Almost 70 percent of the recipients were dead within four months. So, when in the beginning of 1969 a German transplant team in Munich under the auspices of Rudolf Zenker finally decided to transplant a heart,[45] the actual number of transplantations was already diminishing because of the bad long-term results.[46] The two German transplantations in February and in March 1969 failed like many others before. Nevertheless, the public was satisfied that German medical science was up to international standards.[47] A scandal arose, however, because journalists found out the name of the donors in these cases and had molested shamelessly their families at the funeral and at home.[48] The president of the *Hartmannbund*, an important medical professional organisation, blamed Zenker for not protecting the integrity of the donor's family and violating professional discretion.[49] There was an imminent threat that the public would change its mind about heart transplantation if the medical profession did not confirm its willingness to respect and protect the interests of the both the donor and the recipient and their families. In August 1969 Barnard's second transplant patient Philip Blaiberg died from chronic rejection. He had been one of the rare long-term survivors. His death showed that heart transplantation was still a hazardous task which medicine was not really prepared for. A moratorium on heart transplantation ensued which lasted for the next ten years. Nearly all transplantation teams abandoned the technique.[50]

In spite of these difficulties brain death remained uncontested. The concept of brain death had been popularised efficiently and was accepted by lawyers as a scientific necessity and a tribute to modernity. The competency of physicians to determine the essence of death had been established. No formal procedure to obtain consent for the donation of organs had been defined and senior lawyers and theologians had expressed their conviction that consent was neither legally nor morally required.[51] Nevertheless, Zenker declared that in any case he would abstain from explanting organs without explicit consent from the donor or his proxies.[52] The concept of brain death relied on a tacit agreement that should better not be disturbed by a disrespectful treatment of the patients involved.[53] In the following thirty years, several attempts were made to implement the concept of brain death legally. But this last task proved to be rather difficult. In the late sixties and early seventies lawyers voted against a formal inclusion of brain death in German law because medical science must first develop exact criteria for the determination of brain death. In fact, the moratorium on heart transplantation diminished the practical need for legal certainty. But, during the seventies kidney explantation from brain dead donors became more and more common. Whereas before 1967 kidneys had been explanted from either living related donors or non-heart-beating cadavers, they could now also be procured from brain dead heart-beating donors.[54] Moreover, in 1978 the drug cyclosporin A was shown to significantly reduce immunological reactions in organ transplantation. Surgeons from Stanford University, USA, published encouraging results in heart transplantation.[55]

In 1978 the German federal government promoted a transplantation bill for parliamentary discussion.[56] The bill did not mention a definition of death but left this entirely to the medical profession. As the Minister of Justice, the Social Democrat Hans-Jochen Vogel, confirmed, the concept of brain death was not controversial at all.[57] But the political parties were not able to come to an agreement over consent procedures. The governing Social Democrats voted for the right to explant organs when the donor had not explicitly dissented during her or his lifetime.[58] However, the Federal Medical Association was not convinced that this solution would in fact serve their needs.[59] One of the leading transplant surgeons, Rudolf Pichlmayr, said that he was afraid of adverse reactions from the public that could negatively affect transplantation surgery.[60] In March 1980 the Minister of Justice abandoned his initiative and recommended a period of further reflections on the issue.

Nevertheless, one year later the first German heart transplantation after the moratorium was performed in Munich.[61] In 1982 a scientific committee of the German Federal Medical Association issued its first official statement on the concept of brain death and the criteria for determining it. In accordance with the opinion of the Ministry of Justice the committee claimed the determination of death to be a purely scientific task. It confirmed brain death to be the scientific equivalent of the death of a human being. The language of the statement was now that of the exact sciences: 'Brain death is the death of a human being.' 'The list of prerequisites and criteria for the determination of brain death [...] correspond to the present state of scientific knowledge.'[62] 13 out of 16 members of the committee were physicians, the remaining three being the judicial counsellor of the Federal Medical Association, a lawyer and the moral theologian Franz Böckle. Public opinion at that time was in favour of transplantation.[63] Television stars publicly supported organ donation. However, for many people a slight unease prevailed that somebody was called dead whose heart was still beating regularly. But, as *Der Spiegel* reassured its readers, this was 'but a fictitious paradox'.[64] Although, by this time, it must have become clear that the first heart transplantation had been a fatal experiment doomed to fail because of the well-known immunological problems, *Der Spiegel* was still an enthusiastic admirer of Christiaan Barnard. In 1983, when Barnard left his position at the Grote Schuur Hospital the news magazine complimented him on being the 'first physician to dare to transplant the still twitching heart of a dead woman' and who 'surprised again and again with new variants of his

art of healing'.[65] Nevertheless the belief in the blessings of science was
gradually undermined. The instrumental rationality of simple modernisation
demanded that setbacks should be answered with an intensified effort to
reach the intended aim and that side effects were but the price to pay for
scientific progress. In simple modernity the concept of brain death was
an inevitable side effect of technical progress in intensive care medicine
and transplantation techniques. The difficulties in determining consent
procedures would be likewise interpreted as the result of man's failure to
accept the rational consequences of ongoing medical progress. Taking these
side effects for serious problems implied being in opposition to a thoroughly
logical and necessary development.

In reflexive modernity, however, side effects and risks are treated no
longer as an inevitable tribute to modernisation. Instead they can contradict
the supremacy of instrumental rationality. In reflexive modernity questions
arise such as: which risks do we really have to or want to live with? Who is
defining which risks are negligible? Who is going to control the side effects
of scientific knowledge and technological applications? Risk management
becomes an eminently political question. In risk society it is usually not the
big political parties who take up the issue but small action groups with no
definite political programme, a result of an ongoing individualisation of
society in the process of disembedding social structures. This entails a new
conception of politics which Beck calls 'sub-politics', political activity
driven by individuals and social groups outside the political parties and
other corporative institutions.[66] Action groups are contesting scientific
competence to define what is rational and which risks are to be tolerated.
They contribute to the demonopolisation of 'institutionalised' scientists
since they make use of scientific counter expertise to defend their dissenting
views.[67]

During the eighties the social risks of medical science became
highly disputed. The social costs of *in vitro* fertilisation or gene technology
seemed to outweigh future merits. The increase in organ transplantation
engendered a commercialised organ trade from underdeveloped to highly
developed countries.[68] This sad reality nurtured fantasies about people being
kidnapped solely for the purpose of keeping their bodies alive in commercial
organ banks. The renowned German gynaecologist Fritz K. Beller caused a
public scandal when he proposed that encephalic newborns should be used
as organ donors.[69] When, in fact, in 1967 Kantrowitz had used the heart of
an anencephalic for the first heart transplantation in the United States, this
fact had gone rather unnoticed in Germany.[70] The worst fantasies about dead
being kept 'alive' on medical devices seemed to come true in 1992. On

5 October, the 18-year-old Marion Ploch was severely brain injured in a car accident and was delivered to Erlangen University Hospital. She was 13 weeks pregnant. The young women was soon declared brain dead and the parents were asked for permission to explant organs. But the father of Marion Ploch distrusted the concept of brain death. Desperately, he asked a German mass circulation newspaper for help. In the meantime the surgeons responsible had changed their mind and were now determined to maintain the pregnancy. Although the parents wished their daughter could die in dignity they did not dare to protest.[71] The news of the 'baby of the pregnant cadaver' and the dispute between parents and physicians spread rapidly through the media. The public was scandalised. In fact, this shock eventually jeopardised the tacit agreement on the use of the concept of brain death. Firstly, it strongly contradicted popular beliefs about the essence of death. How could a dead person be pregnant and give birth to a child? Secondly, confidence that brain death would not be used against the interests of the dead and his or her proxies was shattered. This time physicians had declared in public that the proxies' wishes were not relevant in this case.[72]

Since 1992, several newspapers have resumed the discussion about the validity of the concept of brain death. The German weekly *Die Zeit* published a series of articles on the relevance of brain death.[73] Even *Der Spiegel* abandoned its scientific optimism and became one of the leading print media to attack scientific claims on brain death.[74] Several action groups issued critical statements on maintaining pregnancy in the event of brain death. When, in 1994, the governing Social Democrats in the federal state of Rhineland-Palatine passed a transplantation bill that recognised brain death and the so-called 'dissent solution' as the consent procedure, the public uproar was immense. The Prime Minister of Rhineland-Palatine was forced to withdraw the bill.[75] A parliamentary initiative to pass a nationwide transplantation law has been confronted with similar difficulties.[76] The criticism has more focused on the determination of death.[77] Members of action groups, physicians, theologians, philosophers, and lawyers expressed their doubt that brain death could be equated with human death.[78] On 25 June 1997 about thirty percent of the members of the *Bundestag* voted against the legal implementation of brain death as the death of a person.[79]

The arguments for and against brain death are still the same as in the sixties and seventies. What has definitely changed is the belief in the natural supremacy of scientific expertise. The definition of death has become a matter of 'sub-politics'. Beck's categories of simple and reflexive modernisation help to explain how different social actors such as physicians, theologians, lawyers, politicians or the media dealt with the new way of treating the dead or supposed-to-be dead in different periods. The social consensus on modernisation that once allowed systematic misunderstandings of the nature of the concept of brain death to be ignored has now broken down. Whereas in simple modernity the new concept of death was considered but a minor side effect of medical progress, it has now become a risk of scientific development that has to be managed politically and is being used to regain social control over medical science.

# Notes

1 *Der Spiegel*, No. 7 (1994), 162. Quotations from German publications have been translated by the author.

2 *Der Spiegel*, No. 10 (1997), 228.

3 U. Beck, *Risikogesellschaft. Auf dem Weg in eine andere Moderne* (Frankfurt/M., 1986), Engl. translation: *Risk Society: Towards a New Modernity* (London, 1992). U. Beck, *Die Erfindung des Politischen. Zu einer Theorie reflexiver Modernisierung* (Frankfurt/M., 1993). U. Beck, 'The Reinvention of Politics: Towards a Theory of Reflexive Modernization' in U. Beck, A. Giddens & S. Lash (eds), *Reflexive Modernization. Politics, Tradition and Aesthetics in the Modern Social Order* (Cambridge, 1994), 1–55.

4 Beck, 'Reflexive Modernization', 2.

5 Beck, 'Reflexive Modernization', 3.

6 P. Mollaret, M. Goulon, 'Le coma dépassé (mémoire préliminaire)', *Revue neurologique*, 101/1 (1959), 3–15. P. Mollaret, 'Über die äussersten Möglichkeiten der Wiederbelebung. Die Grenzen zwischen Leben und Tod', *Münchener medizinische Wochenschrift*, 104 (1962), 1539–45. Mollaret, who is cited usually as the first to equate brain death with the death of a human being, was rather reluctant, in fact, to accept a new definition of death. See also R.A. Frowein, K.H. Euler & A. Karim-Nejad, 'Grenzen der Wiederbelebung bei schweren Hirntraumen', *Langenbecks Archiv für klinische Chirurgie*, 308 (1964), 276–81. W. Laves, 'Agonie', *Münchener medizinische Wochenschrift*, 107 (1965), 113–18. W. Spann, 'Strafrechtliche Probleme an der Grenze von Leben und Tod', *Deutsche Zeitschrift für die gesamte gerichtliche Medizin*, 57 (1966), 26–30. W. Spann & E.W. Liebhardt, 'Reanimation und Feststellung des Todeszeitpunktes', *Münchener medizinische Wochenschrift*, 108 (1966), 1410–14. W. Spann, J. Kugler & E.W. Liebhardt, 'Tod und elektrische Stille im EEG', *Münchener medizinische Wochenschrift*, 42 (1967), 2161–67. A short description of the early history of the notion of brain death, from a medical point of view, can be found in H. Schneider, 'Der Hirntod. Begriffsgeschichte und Pathogenese', *Der Nervenarzt*, 41 (1970), 381–87, 381. For a history of attitudes towards the notion of death see M.S. Pernick, 'Back From the Grave: Recurring Controversies Over Defining and Diagnosing Death in History' in R.M. Zaner (ed.), *Death: Beyond Whole-brain Criteria* (Dordrecht, 1988), 17–74. H.-M. Culmann, *Zur geschichtlichen Entwicklung der Todesauffassung des Arztes im europäischen Raum* (Diss. med. Freiburg, 1986).

7 W. Brosig & R. Nagel, *Nierentransplantation* (Berlin, 1965). K.H. Bauer, 'Über Rechtsfragen bei homologer Organtransplantation aus der Sicht des Klinikers (unter besonderer Berücksichtigung der Krebsübertragung)', *Der Chirurg*, 38 (1967), 245–51. K.E. Seiffert, 'Überblick über den gegenwärtigen Stand der Transplantation von Organen und Geweben', *Der Chirurg*, 38 (1967), 255–59. D. Kirchheim & R.D. Robertson, 'Biologische Grundlagen und Fortschritte in der Nierentransplantation. II. Patienten- und Spenderwahl, Organkonservierung', *Der*

*Urologe*, 6 (1967), 67–74. For the history of kidney transplantation see F. Largiadèr, 'History of Organ Transplantation' in F. Largiadèr (ed.), *Organ Transplantation* (Stuttgart, 1970), 2–12. F.D. Moore, *Transplantation* (Philadelphia, London, 1963), German translation with introduction by W. Brendel (Berlin, Heidelberg, 1970). For the early history of organ transplantation see T. Schlich, *Die Erfindung der Organtransplantation. Erfolg und Scheitern des chirurgischen Organersatzes (1880– 1930)* (Frankfurt, New York, 1998). See also T. Schlich, 'Medizingeschichte und Ethik der Transplantationsmedizin: Die Erfindung der Organtransplantation' in F.W. Albert, W. Land & E. Zwierlein (eds), *Transplantationsmedizin und Ethik. Auf dem Weg zu einem gesellschaftlichen Konsens* (Lengerich, Berlin, 1994), 11–32.

8    E.W. Liebhardt, 'Zivilrechtliche Probleme an der Grenze zwischen Leben und Tod', *Deutsche Zeitschrift für die gesamte gerichtliche Medizin*, 57 (1966), 31–36. G. Kaiser, 'Künstliche Insemination und Transplantation. Juristische und rechtspolitische Probleme' in H. Göppinger (ed.), *Arzt und Recht. Medizinisch-juristische Grenzprobleme unserer Zeit* (Munich, 1966), 58–95. K. Engisch, 'Über Rechtsfragen bei homologer Organtransplantation. Ergänzende Bemerkungen aus der Sicht des Juristen (des Kriminalisten)', *Der Chirurg*, 38 (1967), 252–55.

9    M. Bos, *The Diffusion of Heart and Liver Transplantation Across Europe* (London, 1991), 15–21, 42–48. W. Brendel, 'Anhang. Entwicklung und Ergebnisse seit 1963' in Moore (ed.), *Transplantation*, 159–89. T. Schlich, 'Die Geschichte der Herztransplantation. Chirurgie, Wissenschaft, Ethik' in A. Frewer, M. Köhler & C. Rödel (eds), *Herztransplantation und Ethik. Historische und philosophische Aspekte eines paradigmatischen Eingriffs der modernen Medizin* (Erlanger Studien zur Ethik in der Medizin, Bd. 4) (Erlangen, Jena, 1996), 13–38. T. Stark, *Knife to the Heart: the Story of Transplant Surgery* (London, 1996). For a sociological view see R.C. Fox & J.P. Swazey, *The Courage to Fail. A Social View of Organ Transplants and Dialysis* (Chicago, London, 1974).

10    *Der Spiegel*, No. 12 (1968), 120.

11    *Die Welt*, No. 282 (1967), 1.

12    *Der Spiegel*, No. 51 (1967), 154.

13    *Frankfurter Allgemeine Zeitung*, No. 298, 13 December 1967, 7. Only the editors of the Bavarian newspaper *Süddeutsche Zeitung*, Christian Schütze and Otmar Katz, remained sceptical in the beginning. See e.g. C. Schütze, 'Herzchirurgie mit offenen Fragen', *Süddeutsche Zeitung*, No. 12, 13/14 January 1968, 13; O. Katz, 'Erst das Skalpell, dann die Moral', *Süddeutsche Zeitung*, No. 26, 30 January 1968, 8. In 1969, when Munich became the first German town where a cardiac transplantation took place, this critical attitude had changed into an optimism about the results of medical progress. See e.g. G. Sittner, 'Wir werden keine Jagd auf Spender machen', *Süddeutsche Zeitung*, No. 40, 15/16 February 1969, 3; G. Sittner, 'Am Blutpfropf scheiterte die Verpflanzung', *Süddeutsche Zeitung*, No. 41, 17 February 1969, 3.

14    G. Schettler, H. Gillmann, E. Ritz et al., 'Indikationen und Kontraindikationen der Organtransplantation', *Studium Generale*, 23 (1970), 301–12, 303. E.-W. Hanack,

'Rechtsprobleme bei Organtransplantationen', *Studium Generale*, 23 (1970), 428–43, 429.

15 *Frankfurter Allgemeine Zeitung*, No. 26, 31 January 1968, Natur und Wissenschaft. See also the commentary on the first German heart transplantation by F. Deich in *Die Welt*, No. 40, 17 February 1969, 2.

16 *Die Welt*, No. 298, 22 December 1967, 2.

17 M. Malan, '"Herrgott, es schlägt wieder". Die Herzverpflanzungen des Professor Barnard', *Der Spiegel*, No. 13 (1968), 109–22, 109. See also *Frankfurter Allgemeine Zeitung*, No. 302, 30 December 1967, 18.

18 *Die Welt*, No. 298, 22 December 1967, 2.

19 *Die Welt*, No. 38, 14 February 1968, 7. According to Kautzky the hypothesis that death and brain death are identical was neither provable nor practically adequate. The vice president of the German Society of Surgery, W. Wachsmuth, publicly warned against hastening the death of a patient by removing his organs. *Die Welt*, No. 13, 16 January 1968, 2. A determined critic of the equation of brain death and death was the Würzburg neurosurgeon J. Gerlach. J. Gerlach, 'Syndrome des Sterbens und der Vita reducta', *Münchener medizinische Wochenschrift*, 111 (1969), 169–76. J. Gerlach, 'Gehirntod und totaler Tod', *Münchener medizinische Wochenschrift*, 111 (1969), 732–36. J. Gerlach, 'Bedeutet Gehirntod auch menschlichen Tod?', *Fortschritte der Medizin*, 88 (1970), 399–400, 444.

20 *Frankfurter Allgemeine Zeitung*, No. 2, 3 January 1968, 7.

21 *Der Spiegel*, No. 2 (1968), 74. Italics by the author.

22 But Zenker expressed his belief that the surgical venture was legally and morally justifiable. *Frankfurter Allgemeine Zeitung*, No. 295, 20 December 1967, 8. See also R. Zenker & H. Pichlmaier, 'Organverpflanzung beim Menschen', *Deutsche medizinische Wochenschrift*, 93 (1968), 713–20.

23 *Frankfurter Allgemeine Zeitung*, No. 2, 3 January 1968, 18.

24 *Der Spiegel*, No. 2 (1968), 72.

25 *Der Spiegel*, No. 10 (1968), 5 (editorial).

26 *Der Spiegel*, No. 7 (1968), 119f.

27 See also one from a series of articles about the future of German universities. *Der Spiegel*, No. 30 (1969), 86–95, especially pp. 86, 94.

28 F. Böckle at a round table discussion during the annual meeting of the German Society of Neurosurgery. 'Der zentrale Atemstillstand, eine ärztliche Konflikt-situation (Podiumsdiskussion, gehalten am 20. 6. 1968 auf der Jahrestagung der Deutschen Gesellschaft für Neurochirurgie in Göttingen)' in K.-A. Bushe (ed.), *Fortschritte auf dem Gebiet der Neurochirurgie* (Stuttgart, 1970), 38–58, 45.

29 H. Thielecke, *Wer darf leben? Ethische Probleme der modernen Medizin* (Munich, 1970), 38f.

30 H. Thielecke, 'Das Recht des Menschen auf seinen Tod', *Fortschritte der Medizin*, 86 (1968), 1067–68.

31 Reported in *Die Welt*, No. 128, 4 June 1968, 10. The theologian M. Honecker from Bonn University also declared that it was a task of medicine to define the criteria of death. M. Honecker, 'Freiheit, den Tod anzunehmen. Theologische Gedanken aus Anlass der Organtransplantationen' in M. Honecker (ed.), *Aspekte und Probleme der Organverpflanzung* (Neukirchen-Vluyn, 1973), 183–203, 192. See also W. Ruff, *Organverpflanzung. Ethische Probleme aus katholischer Sicht* (Munich, 1971). The Catholic theologians K. Rahner and J. Gründel also accepted the thesis that brain death equated with death. K. Rahner, 'Theologische Erwägungen über den Eintritt des Todes' in K. Rahner, *Schriften zur Theologie*. Vol. IX, 2nd edn (Einsiedeln, Zürich, Köln, 1972), 323–35, 327. J. Gründel, 'Der relative Wert irdisch leiblichen menschlichen Lebens und der Tod aus theologischer Perspektive' in W. Krösl & E. Scherzer (eds), *Die Bestimmung des Todeszeitpunktes. Kongress in der Wiener Hofburg vom 4. bis 6. Mai 1972* (Vienna, 1973), 321–27. The Protestant theologian D. Walther, however, hold a different position. He was sceptical whether medical science could decide on these questions with scientific objectivity at all. D. Walther, 'Theologisch-ethische Aspekte einer Herztransplantation' in Honecker (ed.), *Aspekte und Probleme der Organverpflanzung*, 19–32, 20f. The moral theologian H. Pompey from Würzburg was also opposed to the new definition of death (but not to heart explantation from irreversibly comatose patients). He seems to have been strongly influenced by the Würzburg neurosurgeon J. Gerlach, a critic of the brain death definition. H. Pompey, 'Gehirntod und totaler Tod. Moraltheologische Erwägungen zur Herztransplantation', *Münchener medizinische Wochenschrift*, 111 (1969), 736–41.

32 E.-W. Hanack, 'Todeszeitbestimmung, Reanimation und Organtransplantation', *Deutsches Ärzteblatt*, 66/19 (1969), 1320–31, 1320. See also Hanack, 'Rechtsprobleme bei Organtransplantationen', 432. The Attorney of the German Federal Supreme Court (*Bundesanwalt*), M. Kohlhaas, complained that physicians wanted to defer the determination of death to the lawyers. M. Kohlhaas, 'Zur Feststellung des Todeszeitpunktes Verstorbener', *Deutsche medizinische Wochenschrift*, 93 (1968), 412–14, 413f. See also P. Bockelmann, 'Strafrechtliche Aspekte der Organtransplantation (85. Tagung der Deutschen Gesellschaft für Chirurgie vom 17. bis 20. April 1968)', *Langenbecks Archiv für klinische Chirurgie*, 322 (1968), 44–60, 53. Only the lawyer G. Geilen questioned the normative competence of medical science in this special case. G. Geilen, 'Das Leben des Menschen in den Grenzen des Rechts. Zu den Wandlungen des Todesbegriffs und zu neuen Schutzproblemen des werdenden Lebens', *Zeitschrift für das gesamte Familienrecht*, 15 (1968), 121–30, 124f.

33 *Die Welt*, No. 38, 14 January 1968, 7.

34 See, for example, the statements of the neurosurgeon J. Gerlach, at the discussion in Bonn, December 1968, published in H. Penin & C. Käufer (eds), *Der Hirntod. Todeszeitbestimmung bei irreversiblem Funktionsverlust des Gehirns* (Stuttgart, 1969),

44f, 53f. See also 'Der zentrale Atemstillstand... (Podiumsdiskussion)' in Bushe (ed.), *Fortschritte*, 38–58, especially the statement of the Protestant theologian W. Trillhaas, p. 46. The neurosurgeon R. Kautzky said it was peculiar how every discipline tried to defer the decision, p. 44. See also E. Heinitz, *Rechtliche Fragen der Organtransplantation* (Berlin, 1970).

35  Penin & Käufer (eds), *Der Hirntod*, 106–134 (discussion III). J. Wawersik, 'Kriterien des Todes', *Studium Generale*, 23 (1970), 319–30, 325. A. Gütgemann & C. Käufer, 'Organentnahme und Transplantation', *Deutsche medizinische Wochenschrift*, 96 (1971), 609–14, 611.

36  Zenker & Pichlmaier, 'Organverpflanzung', 716. H. Kress, *Ärztliche Fragen bei der Organtransplantation* (Berlin, 1970), 8. The lawyer P. Bockelmann complained about this diagnostic uncertainty. He maintained that organs should not be removed until cardiac and respiratory arrest had definitely proven the donor's death. Nevertheless, he did not object to the brain death definition as such. Bockelmann, 'Strafrechtliche Aspekte der Organtransplantation', 55f.

37  Social acceptance and practical aspects of diagnostic instruments played an important role in determining the diagnostic procedure. C. Wiesemann, 'Instrumentalisierte Instrumente: EEG, zerebrale Angiographie und die Etablierung des Hirntod-Konzepts' in C. Meinel (ed.), *Instrument – Experiment* (forthcoming).

38  E.g. Kohlhaas, 'Zur Feststellung des Todeszeitpunktes', 414.

39  Kress, *Ärztliche Fragen bei der Organtransplantation*, 6. See also O. Pribilla, 'Juristische, ärztliche und ethische Fragen zur Todesfeststellung', *Deutsches Ärzteblatt*, 65/41 (1968), 2256–59, 2318–22, 2396–98, 2397. During a discussion at an international conference in Vienna, W. Spann, professor of forensic medicine at Freiburg University, went so far as to say: 'Ladies and gentlemen, the determination of death is a task of the general public or society. I personally have expressed the opinion that there is and there will be no way to determine the time of death by scientific methods.' 'Allgemeine Diskussion' in Krösl & Scherzer (eds), *Die Bestimmung des Todeszeitpunktes*, 339–62, 349. The 'general public', at this conference represented by the journalist T. Chorherr, immediately rejected this suggestion, p. 359. See also the statement of W. Kramer, a neurologist from Leiden university clinic, pp. 349, 357. The normative aspect of the definition of brain death and the need for a social consensus had already been stressed by Spann's assistants Liebhardt and Wuermeling in 1968. E.W. Liebhardt & H.-B. Wuermeling, 'Juristische und medizinisch-naturwissenschaftliche Begriffsbildung und die Feststellung des Todeszeitpunktes', *Münchener medizinische Wochenschrift*, 110 (1968), 1661–65. The dispute about responsibility for defining criteria for human death had already surfaced in the early days of artificial respiration. In 1957, the Austrian anaesthetist B. Haid had asked Pope Pius XII to clarify when a human being on artificial respiration could be considered dead. But the Pope had infallibly referred this problem back to the doctors. S. Schellong, *Künstliche Beatmung. Strukturgeschichte eines ethischen Dilemmas* (Stuttgart, 1990), 145f.

40  Except for the penologist G. Geilen. G. Geilen, 'Medizinischer Fortschritt und juristischer Todesbegriff' in H. Lüttger, H. Blei & P. Hanau (eds), *Festschrift für Ernst Heinitz zum 70. Geburtstag* (Berlin, 1972), 373–96, 392f. G. Geilen, 'Rechtsfragen der Todeszeitbestimmung' in Krösl & Scherzer (eds), *Die Bestimmung des Todeszeitpunktes*, 285–93, 288. G. Geilen, 'Rechtsfragen der Organtransplantation' in Honecker (ed.), *Aspekte und Probleme der Organtransplantation*, 179.

41  P. Bockelmann, 'Allgemeine Diskussion' in Krösl & Scherzer (eds), *Die Bestimmung des Todeszeitpunktes*, 339–62, 341.

42  Kommission für Reanimation und Organtransplantation der Deutschen Gesellschaft für Chirurgie, 'Todeszeichen und Todeszeitbestimmung', *Der Chirurg*, 39 (1968), 196–97. English translation in Largiadèr (ed.), *Organ Transplantation*, Appendix 3. Three months later, a statement of a Harvard Medical Committee on brain death was issued (August 1968). Ad Hoc Committee of the Harvard Medical School to Examine the Definition of Brain Death, 'A Definition of Irreversible Coma', *The Journal of the American Medical Association*, 205 (1968), 85–88. H. Jonas' arguments against the Harvard definition of death were not discussed in Germany at that time. B. Weiss, *Rezeption der Einwände von Hans Jonas gegen die Feststellung des Hirntodes als Tod des Menschen* (Diss. med. Erlangen, 1991).

43  This rather nominalistic use of brain death was harshly criticised by G. Geilen, 'Rechtsfragen der Todeszeitbestimmung' in Krösl & Scherzer (eds), *Die Bestimmung des Todeszeitpunktes*, 292, and in 1984 again by the lawyer A. Laufs, 'Juristische Probleme des Hirntodes' in H. Gänshirt, P. Berlit & G. Haack (eds), *Kardiovaskuläre Erkrankungen und Nervensystem, Neurotoxikologie, Probleme des Hirntodes* (Berlin, Heidelberg, 1985), 559–64, 561.

44  *Der Spiegel*, No. 47 (1968), 198, and No. 43 (1969), 202. Bos, *Diffusion of Heart and Liver Transplantation*, 18.

45  The first German patient with a heart transplant, J. Zehner, died one day after the operation. The case was officially published on 4 April 1969 in the *Münchener medizinische Wochenschrift*. R. Zenker, W. Klinner, F. Sebening et al., 'Herztransplantation – Möglichkeiten und Problematik', *Münchener medizinische Wochenschrift*, 111 (1969), 749–54.

46  Bos, *Diffusion of Heart and Liver Transplantation*, 18. Brendel, 'Anhang.' in Moore (ed.), *Transplantation*, 177.

47  *Der Spiegel*, No. 8 (1969), 132f. The headline was 'Heart Transplantations: Lost Years' which implied that German surgeons had hesitated too long.

48  *Die Welt*, No. 70, 24 March 1969, 22. *Der Spiegel*, No. 14 (1969), 82.

49  *Frankfurter Allgemeine Zeitung*, No. 40, 17 February 1969, 8.

50  There had been 151 cardiac transplantations performed through 25 September 1969. J.P. Swazey & R.C. Fox, 'The Clinical Moratorium' in R.C. Fox (ed.), *Essays in Medical Sociology. Journeys into the Field* (New York, 1979), 325–63, 326. However, Swazey and Fox could not find evidence in English publications that Blaiberg's death was directly responsible for the moratorium. Ibid, 326, fn 3. See also

Bos, *Diffusion of Heart and Liver Transplantation*, 18. Schlich, 'Geschichte der Herztransplantation', 23.

51  In 1969, the federal minister of health K. Strobel declared it was the prevailing opinion that hospital physicians were allowed to explant cadaveric organs even against the proxies' wishes. Bundestagsdrucksache 5/4568. See also F. Böckle and the lawyer C. Roxin in 'Der zentrale Atemstillstand... (Podiumsdiskussion)' in Bushe (ed.), *Fortschritte*, 38–58, 57f. F. Böckle, 'Ethische Aspekte der Organ-transplantation beim Menschen', *Studium Generale*, 23 (1970), 444–59, 459. Heinitz, *Rechtliche Fragen der Organtransplantation*, 24. The physician and Catholic theologian W. Ruff even found it permissible to explant organs from the dying. Ruff, *Organverpflanzung*, 149. The lawyer H. Trockel maintained however that proxy consent should be obtained. H. Trockel, 'Rechtliche Probleme der Organ-transplantation', *Medizinische Klinik*, 64 (1969), 666–68.

52  'IX. Rundgespräch: Atemstillstand – Herzstillstand – Tod. (86. Tagung der Deutschen Gesellschaft für Chirurgie vom 9. bis 12. April 1969)', *Langenbecks Archiv für Chirurgie*, 325 (1968), 1092–99, 1099.

53  However, on 25 February 1970 the County Court of Bonn had ruled in a civil suit that proxy consent was necessary for organ explantation if it could be obtained in reasonable time. Landgericht Bonn, *Urteil vom 25. 2. 1970* (7/O 230/69). The sentence was published in *Juristenzeitung*, 26 (1971), 56–62. It was criticised by the surgeons involved in this case: A. Gütgemann & C. Käufer, 'Organentnahme und Transplantation', *Deutsche medizinische Wochenschrift*, 96 (1971), 609–14, 612f.

54  Bos, *Diffusion of Heart and Liver Transplantation*, 32f.

55  Ibid., 19, 29.

56  'Entwurf eines Gesetzes über Eingriffe an Verstorbenen zu Transplantationszwecken (Transplantationsgesetz)', Bundestagsdrucksache 8/2681, Anlage 1 (final draft from 16 March 1979). For a short history of this bill see W. Höfling & S. Rixen, *Verfassungsfragen der Transplantationsmedizin* (Tübingen, 1996), 24–34.

57  H.-J. Vogel, 'Zustimmung oder Widerspruch. Bemerkungen zu einer Kernfrage der Organtransplantation', *Neue juristische Wochenschrift*, 33/12 (1980), 625–29, 626.

58  Nowadays this is called 'dissent solution'. On the other hand, the *Bundesrat*, which at that time was dominated by the Christian Democratic party, voted for a consent solution. The donor should declare during her or his lifetime whether she or he agreed to organ explantation. In case of her or his death proxies could decide in the best interests of the patient. This was intended explicitly to improve the relationship between physicians and proxies. 'Stellungnahme des Bundesrates', Bundestagsdrucksache 1979, 8/2681, Anlage 2, 16.

59  Vogel, 'Zustimmung oder Widerspruch', 629, fn. 19.

60  Pichlmayr was invited as a medical expert to a hearing of the judicial committee (*Rechtsausschuss*) of the *Bundestag*. Höfling & Rixen, *Verfassungsfragen der Transplantationsmedizin*, 33, Fn. 124. Pichlmayr was also cited in *Der Spiegel*, No. 50 (1983), 102.

61 The operation was performed on 19 August 1981. P. Überfuhr, B. Reichart, A. Welz et al., 'Bericht über eine erfolgreiche orthotope Herztransplantation in Deutschland', *Klinische Wochenschrift*, 60 (1982), 1435–42. This time the public was not informed until the patient was definitely out of danger. From August 1981 to February 1983 seven successful heart transplantations were performed in Munich. *Der Spiegel*, No. 8 (1983), 207f.

62 The committee was founded in November 1979. A short resumé of its deliberations was published in the *Deutsche Ärzteblatt*: Wissenschaftlicher Beirat der Bundesärztekammer, 'Kriterien des Hirntodes. Entscheidungshilfen zur Feststellung des Hirntodes', *Deutsches Ärzteblatt*, 79 (1982), (C)35–41, 35, 38. Unfortunately, I could not get permission to see the archive of the 'Wissenschaftlicher Beirat'.

63 The official commentary on the transplantation bill of the *Bundesregierung* from 1979 stated that even from a medical point of view it was not necessary to allow organ explantation against the explicit will of the brain dead because public support for transplantation was ever increasing. 'Entwurf eines Gesetzes über Eingriffe an Verstorbenen zu Transplantationszwecken (Transplantationsgesetz)', Bundestagsdrucksache 8/2681, 6.

64 *Der Spiegel*, No. 50 (1983), 102.

65 *Der Spiegel*, No. 32 (1983), 145.

66 Beck, *Erfindung des Politischen*, 149–63. See also A. Giddens, 'Living in a Post-Traditional Society' in Beck, Giddens & Lash (eds), *Reflexive Modernization*, 56–109.

67 Beck, *Risikogesellschaft*, 255–68. See also C. Wiesemann, 'Medizin und reflexive Modernisierung am Beispiel der Hirntod-Kontroverse' in R. Hohlfeld & C. Lau (eds), *Wissenschaft und reflexive Modernisierung* (Finck, 1998, in press).

68 For the first time in 1986, the member of the *Bundestag* Emmerlich (SPD) demanded a political reaction to the commercialised organ trade. Question to the Federal Government, 10 October 1986, Bundestagsdrucksache 10/6207. Since 1988, members of the Green Party regularly addressed subjects like the organ trade, 'Baby Fae', or brain death in parliament. Bundestagsdrucksachen 11/5163 and 5165–68.

69 F.K. Beller & J. Reeve, 'Brain life and brain death – the anencephalic as an explanatory example. A contribution to transplantation', *The Journal of Medicine and Philosophy*, 14 (1989), 5–23. H.-B. Wuermeling, 'Gefährliches Nachdenken über anencephale Neugeborene als Organspender', *Medizinische Ethik. Sonderbeilage des Ärzteblatt Baden-Württemberg*, 4/27 (1988).

70 Bos, *Diffusion of Heart and Liver Transplantation*, 17.

71 This interpretation of the events was maintained by the parents after the spontaneous abortion of the foetus on 11 November 1992. See the presentation of the case from the perspective of M. Ploch's parents in the magazine *Stern*. 'Das darf nie wieder passieren', *Stern*, No. 49 (1992), 220f. See also 'Leben in der Leiche', *Der Spiegel*, No. 43 (1992), 320–25. For a discussion of the case from an academic

point of view see G. Bockenheimer-Lucius & E. Seidler (eds), *Hirntod und Schwangerschaft. Dokumentation einer Diskussionsveranstaltung der Akademie für Ethik in der Medizin zum 'Erlanger Fall'* (Stuttgart, 1993). C. Anstötz, 'A Report from Germany. Should a Brain-Dead Pregnant Woman Carry Her Child to Full Term? The Case of the "Erlanger Baby"', *Bioethics*, 7 (1993), 340–50.

72 *Die Zeit*, No. 45, 30 October 1992, 17. See also the statements of I. Retzlaff and H.-B. Wuermeling in Bockenheimer-Lucius & Seidler (eds), *Hirntod und Schwangerschaft*, 32f.

73 See, for example, J. Hoff & J. in der Schmitten, 'Tot?', *Die Zeit*, No. 47 (1992), 56. J. Hoff & J. in der Schmitten, 'Organspende – nur über meine Leiche?', *Die Zeit*, No. 7 (1993), 40.

74 'Im Vorzimmer des Todes', *Der Spiegel*, No. 24 (1994), 212–16. 'Kannibalen am Leichnam?', *Der Spiegel*, No. 7 (1995), 162f. 'Im Grenzland des Todes', *Der Spiegel*, No. 10 (1997), 228–39.

75 *Der Spiegel*, No. 29 (1994), 38.

76 Höfling & Rixen, *Verfassungsfragen der Transplantationsmedizin*, 34–39.

77 See, for example, the transplantation bill proposed by members of the party 'Bündnis 90/Die Grünen' in November 1995 which assumed that a social consensus on the nature of death could not be achieved and that the medical profession had no special privilege to define the essence of death. 'Entwurf eines Gesetzes über die Spende, die Entnahme und die Übertragung von Organen (Transplantationsgesetz – TPG)', 7 November 1995, Bundestagsdrucksache 13/2926, especially p. 11. See also D.B. Linke, 'Die dritte kopernikanische Wende. Transplantationsmedizin und personale Identität', *Ethica*, 1 (1993), 53–64. J. Hoff & J. in der Schmitten (eds), *Wann ist der Mensch tot? Organverpflanzung und Hirntodkriterium* (Reinbek, 1994). P. Bavastro (ed.), *Organspende – der umkämpfte Tod. Gewissensentscheidung angesichts des Sterbens* (Stuttgart, 1995). C. Wiesemann, 'Hirntod und Gesellschaft. Argumente für einen pragmatischen Skeptizismus', *Ethik in der Medizin*, 6 (1995), 16–28. J. Vollmann, 'Medizinische Probleme des Hirntodkriteriums', *Medizinische Klinik*, 91 (1996), 39–45. K. Stapenhorst, 'Über die biologisch-naturwissenschaftlich unzulässige Gleichsetzung von Hirntod und Individualtod und ihre Folgen für die Medizin', *Ethik in der Medizin*, 8 (1996), 79–98. C. Breuer, 'Wann ist der Mensch tot? Der Tod des Menschen in der Auseinandersetzung um die Verwertung seines Körpers', *Zeitschrift für Medizinische Ethik*, 42 (1996), 91–102.

78 H.-U. Gallwas, G. Geilen, L. Geisler et al., 'Wissenschaftler für ein tragfähiges Transplantationsgesetz', *Zeitschrift für Allgemeinmedizin*, 71 (1995), 1109–12. G. Klinkhammer, 'Diskussion um das Transplantationsgesetz. Wann ist der Mensch tot?', *Deutsches Ärzteblatt*, 94/10 (1997), (C)430–32. M. Emmrich, 'Hirntod und Organtransplantation. Debatte im Bundestag über das neue Organtransplantationsgesetz', *Dr. med. Mabuse*, 106, March/April (1997), 22–24.

79 Gesetz über die Spende, Entnahme und Übertragung von Organen (Transplantationsgesetz), Bundestagsdrucksache 13/8027.

# Consolidated Bibliography

Abrams, Lynn & Harvey, Elizabeth (eds.), *Gender Relations in German History* (London, 1996).

Ackerknecht, E.H., 'Legal Medicine in Transition (16th–18th Centuries)', *The Ciba Symposia*, 9 (1950–51), 1286–1304.

Ackerknecht, E.H., *Rudolf Virchow. Arzt, Politiker, Anthropologe* (Stuttgart, 1957).

Ackerknecht, E.H., *Medicine at the Paris Hospital, 1794–1848* (Baltimore, 1967).

Ad Hoc Committee of the Harvard Medical School to Examine the Definition of Brain Death, 'A Definition of Irreversible Coma', *The Journal of the American Medical Association*, 205 (1968), 85–88.

*Akte betr. Sektionen. Leichenmangel (1934–1946)*, Universitätsarchiv der Humboldt-Universität Berlin, Medizinische Fakultät, Dekanat, Nr.281.

Albert, F.W., Land, W. & Zwierlein, W.E. (eds.), *Transplantationsmedizin und Ethik. Auf dem Weg zu einem gesellschaftlichen Konsens* (Berlin, 1994).

Alcalá, Angel (ed.), *The Spanish Inquisition and inquisitorial mind* (Boulder, 1987).

Alexiou, Margaret, *The Ritual Lament in Greek Tradition* (Cambridge, 1974).

*Algemeen Handelsblad*.

Aly, Götz, 'Der saubere und der schmutzige Fortschritt' in Bleker, Johanna & Jachertz, Norbert (eds.), *Reform und Gewissen. "Euthanasie" im Dienst des Fortschritts* (Beiträge zur nationalsozialistischen Gesundheits- und Sozialpolitik 2) (Berlin, 1985), 9–78.

Annas, G.J., *The Nazi Doctors and the Nuremberg Code: Human Rights in Human Experimentation* (New York, 1992).

Anstötz, C., 'A Report from Germany. Should a Brain-Dead Pregnant Woman Carry Her Child to Full Term? The Case of the "Erlanger Baby"', *Bioethics*, 7 (1993), 340–50.

Apollinaire, Guillaume, *L'Oeuvre du marquis de Sade* (Paris, 1909).

Apter, Emily, *Feminizing the Fetish: Psychoanalysis and Narrative Obsession in Turn-of-the-Century France* (Ithaca, 1991).

Arbeitsgruppe zur Erforschung der Geschichte der Karl-Bonhoeffer-Nervenklinik (scientific adviser Aly, Götz) (eds.), *Totgeschwiegen 1933–1945. Zur Geschichte der Wittenauer Heilstätten. Seit 1957 Karl-Bonhoeffer-Nervenklinik* (Berlin, 1989).

Aschoff, Ludwig, 'Über die Bedeutung der Leichenöffnungen und des Tierexperiments für die Volksgesundheit und die soziale Wohlfahrtspflege' in *Wissenschaft und Werktätiges Volk* (Verlag der Notgemeinschaft der Deutschen Wissenschaft), 151–85.

Aschoff, Ludwig, *Ein Gelehrtenleben in Briefen an die Familie* (Freiburg i.Br., 1966).

Aschoff, Ludwig, *Wissenschaft und Werktätiges Volk* (Verlag der Notgemeinschaft der Deutschen Wissenschaft).

Association for Moral and Social Hygiene (ed.), *Regulation 33B. The Medical Aspect, the Legal Aspect, the Social Aspect* (London, 1943).

Augustin, F.L., *Die Königlich preußische Medicinalverfassung, oder vollständige Darstellung aller, das Medicinalwesen und die medcinische Polizei in den Königlich Preußischen Staaten betreffenden Gesetze, Verordnungen und Einrichtungen*, Vol. 4 (Potsdam & Berlin, 1838).

Austoker, J. & Bryder, L. (eds.), *Historical Perspectives on the Role of the MRC* (Oxford, 1989).

Bächtold, Hanns, *Deutscher Soldatenbrauch und Soldatenglaube* (Strasbourg, 1917).

Bächtold-Stäubli, Hanns et al. (eds.), '*Handwörterbuch des Deutschen Aberglaubens*' (*Handwörterbuch zur deutschen Volkskunde, Abt.1: Aberglaube*), Vols. 1–10 (Berlin, 1927–42).

Baker, R., 'Medical Ethics' in Bynum, W.F. & Porter, Roy (eds.), *Companion Encyclopedia of the History of Medicine* (London & New York, 1993), Vol. 2, 852–87.

Ball, Benjamin, *La folie érotique* (Paris, 1888).

Barrows, Susannah, *Distorting Mirrors: Visions of the Crowd in Late Nineteenth-Century France* (New Haven, 1981).

Bauer, Axel, *Die Krankheitslehre auf dem Weg zur naturwissenschaftlichen Morphologie. Pathologie auf den Versammlungen Deutscher Naturforscher und Ärzte von 1822–1872* (Stuttgart, 1989).

Bauer, Hans Georg, *Die Behandlung des menschlichen Leichnams im geltenden deutschen Recht* (Dresden, 1929).

Bauer, K.H., 'Über Rechtsfragen bei homologer Organtransplantation aus der Sicht des Klinikers (unter besonderer Berücksichtigung der Krebsübertragung)', *Der Chirurg*, 38 (1967), 245–51.

Bavastro, P (ed.), *Organspende – der umkämpfte Tod. Gewissensentscheidung angesichts des Sterbens* (Stuttgart, 1995).

Bayer, R. & Gostin, L., 'Legal and Ethical Issues in AIDS' in Gottlieb, M.S. et al., *Current Topics in AIDS, Volume 2* (Chichester, 1989), 263–83.

Bayly, H.W., *Venereal Disease: Its Prevention, Symptoms and Treatment* (London, 1920)

Beardsley, E.H., 'Allied Against Sin. American and British Responses to Venereal Disease in World War I', *Medical History*, 20 (1976), 189–202.

Beck, U., *Risikogesellschaft. Auf dem Weg in eine andere Moderne* (Frankfurt/M., 1986)

Beck, U., *Risk Society: Towards a New Modernity* (London, 1992).

Beck, U., *Die Erfindung des Politischen. Zu einer Theorie reflexiver Modernisierung* (Frankfurt/M., 1993).

Beck, U., 'The Reinvention of Politics: Towards a Theory of Reflexive Modernization' in Beck, U., Giddens, A. & Lash, S. (eds.), *Reflexive Modernization. Politics, Tradition and Aesthetics in the Modern Social Order* (Cambridge, 1994), 1–55.

Beck, U., Giddens, A. & Lash, S. (eds.), *Reflexive Modernization. Politics, Tradition and Aesthetics in the Modern Social Order* (Cambridge, 1994).

Becker, Volker, *Pathologie. Beständigkeit und Wandel* (Berlin & Heidelberg, 1996).

Beinart, J., 'The Inner World of Imperial Sickness: The MRC and Research in Tropical Medicine' in Austoker, J. & Bryder, L. (eds.), *Historical Perspectives on the Role of the MRC* (Oxford, 1989), 109–35.

Beller, F.K. & Reeve, J., 'Brain life and brain death – the anencephalic as an explanatory example. A contribution to transplantation', *The Journal of Medicine and Philosophy*, 14 (1989), 5–23.

Benaroyo, Lazare, 'Pathology and the Crisis of German Medicine (1920–1930): A Study of Ludwig Aschoff's Case' in Prüll, Cay-Rüdiger (with assistance of Woodward, John) (ed.), *Pathology in the 19th and 20th Centuries. The Relationship between Theory and Practice* (Sheffield, 1997), 101–13.

Bennassar, Bartolomé, *L'Inquisition espagnole. XVe–XIXe siècle* (Paris, 1979).

Berard, Alexandre, *La responsibilité morale* (Lyon, 1892).

Berg, M. & Cocks, G. (eds.), *Medicine and Modernity. Public Health and Medical Care in Nineteenth- and Twentieth-Century Germany* (New York & Cambridge, 1997).

Berlinguer, G, *The Human Body. From Slavery to the Biomarket: An Ethical Analysis* (Sheffield, 1999).

Binet, Alfred,'Le fetichisme dans l'amour', *Revue philosophique*, 24 (1887), 143–67, 252–77.

Birkett, Jennifer, *The Sins of the Fathers: Decadence in France, 1870–1914* (London, 1986).

Blackett, B., 'Progress in Social Hygiene 1914–35', *Health & Empire*, New Series, 10 (1935), 179.

Blackett, J.F., 'The Case for the Notification of Venereal Disease', *Medical Officer*, 30 (1923), 193–94.

Bland, L., '"Cleansing the Portals of Life": The Venereal Disease Campaign in the early Twentieth Century', in Langan, M. & Schwarz, B.(eds.), *Crises in the British State, 1880–1930* (London, 1985), 192–208.

Blaschko, Alfred, 'Hygiene der Geschlechtskrankheiten' in Gärtner, A. (ed.), *Weyls Handbuch der Hygiene*, Vol. 8 (Leipzig, 2nd edition 1918–22), 415–16.

Blázquez, Juan, *Madrid. Judíos, herejes y brujas. El tribunal de Corte, 1650–1820* (Toledo, 1990).

Blécourt, Willem de, 'Duivelbanners in de noordelijke Friese Wouden, 1860–1930', *Volkskundig bulletin* 14 (1988), 159–87.

Blécourt, Willem de, 'Het Staphorster boertje. De geneeskundige praktijk van Peter Stegeman (1840–1922)' in Gijswijt-Hofstra, Marijke (ed.), *Geloven in genezen* (Amsterdam, 1991), 171–94.

Blécourt, Willem de, 'Sequah in Amsterdam. Over de invloed van reclame op een medische markt', *Focaal. Tijdschrift voor antropologie* 21 (1993), 131–72.

Blécourt, Willem de, 'Irreguliere genezers in de stad Groningen in de tweede helft van de 19e eeuw', *Gronings Historisch jaarboek* 1 (1994), 126–41.

Blécourt, Willem de, 'Sleeping women; or the awakening of the somnambules', unpublished paper given at the conference *Healing, Magic & Belief*, Woudschoten, 24 September 1994.

Blécourt, Willem de, 'The Tale of Two Brothers. Urine diagnosis and medical politics in the Netherlands and Michigan, early twentieth century', unpublished paper given at the SSHM conference, *Medicine and the Family*, University of Exeter, 1995.

Blécourt, Willem de, 'Cultures of abortion; daily practice in The Hague, early twentieth-century' in Eder, Franz, Hall, Lesley & Hekma, Gert (eds.), *Sexual Cultures in Europe* (Manchester, 1999).

Blécourt, Willem de, *Het Amazonenleger. Irreguliere genezeressen in Nederland, ca. 1850–1930* (Amsterdam, 1999).

Bleker, Johanna, 'Johann Lukas Schönlein (1793–1864)' in Engelhardt, Dietrich v. & Hartmann, Fritz (eds.), *Klassiker der Medizin*, Vol. 2, *Von Philippe Pinel bis Viktor von Weizsäcker* (Munich, 1991), 81–94.

Bleker, Johanna & Jachertz, Norbert (eds.), *Reform und Gewissen. "Euthanasie" im Dienst des Fortschritts* (Beiträge zur nationalsozialistischen Gesundheits und Sozialpolitik 2) (Berlin, 1985).

Bleker, Johanna & Jachertz, Norbert (eds.), *Medizin im "Dritten Reich"* (Cologne, 1993).

Bockelmann, P., 'Strafrechtliche Aspekte der Organtransplantation (85. Tagung der Deutschen Gesellschaft für Chirurgie vom 17. bis 20. April 1968)', *Langenbecks Archiv für klinische Chirurgie*, 322 (1968), 44–60.

Bockelmann, P., 'Allgemeine Diskussion' in Krösl, W. & Scherzer E. (eds.), *Die Bestimmung des Todeszeitpunktes. Kongreß in der Wiener Hofburg vom 4. bis 6. Mai 1972* (Wien, 1973), 339–62.

Bockenheimer Lucius, G. & Seidler, E. (eds.), *Hirntod und Schwangerschaft. Dokumentation einer Diskussionsveranstaltung der Akademie für Ethik in der Medizin zum 'Erlanger Fall'* (Stuttgart, 1993).

Böckle, F. & Roxin, C., 'Der zentrale Atemstillstand, eine ärztliche Konfliktsituation (Podiumsdiskussion, gehalten am 20. 6. 1968 auf der Jahrestagung der Deutschen Gesellschaft für Neurochirurgie in Göttingen)' in Bushe, K.-A. (ed.), *Fortschritte auf dem Gebiet der Neurochirurgie* (Stuttgart, 1970), 38–58.

Böckle, F., 'Ethische Aspekte der Organtransplantation beim Menschen', *Studium Generale*, 23 (1970), 444–59.

Böckle, F., 'Pietät oder Nächstenliebe? Zur sittlichen Bewertung der medizinischen Obduktion', *Der Pathologe*, 4 (1983), 1–2.

Bohne, Gotthold, 'Das Recht zur klinischen Leichensektion' in *Festgabe für Richard Schmidt. Zu seinem siebzigsten Geburtstag am 19. Januar 1932 überreicht von Verehrern und Schülern* (Leipzig, 1932), 105–76.

Bolea, R.C., 'Venereal Diseases in Spain during the last third of the Nineteenth Century: An Approach to the Moral Bases of Public Health', *Dynamis*, 11 (1991) 239–62.

Bond, B. & Roy, I. (eds.), *War and Society. A Yearbook of Military History*, Vol. 2 (London, 1977).

Bond, C. J., 'The Attitude of the State and Society to Anti-Social Diseases', *Health & Empire*, New Series, 1 (1926), 47–48.

Bos, M., *The Diffusion of Heart and Liver Transplantation Across Europe* (London, 1991).

Boyd, K.M., *Scottish Church Attitudes to Sex, Marriage and the Family* (Edinburgh, 1980).

Brandt, A.M., *No Magic Bullet, A Social History of Venereal Disease in the United States since 1880* (Oxford, 1985).

Brandt, A.M., 'Racism and research: the case of the Tuskagee syphilis study' in Leavitt, J.W. & Numbers, R.L., *Sickness and Health in America* (Madison & London, 1985), 331–46.

Brazell, N.E., 'The Significance and Application of Informed Consent', *AORN Journal*, 65 (1997), 377–80, 382, 385–86.

Breitfellner, G., 'Die gesetzliche Sektionspflicht in österreichischen Krankenanstalten', *Der Pathologe*, 7 (1986), 62–63.

Brendel, W., 'Anhang. Entwicklung und Ergebnisse seit 1963' in Moore, F.D. (ed.), *Transplantation. Geschichte und Entwicklung bis zur heutigen Zeit* (Engl. Original Philadelphia & London 1963) (Berlin & Heidelberg, 1970), 159–89.

Breuer, C., 'Wann ist der Mensch tot? Der Tod des Menschen in der Auseinandersetzung um die Verwertung seines Körpers', *Zeitschrift für Medizinische Ethik*, 42 (1996), 91–102.

Bridenthal, Renate, Grossmann, Atina & Kaplan, Marion (eds.), *When Biology Became Destiny* (New York, 1984).

*British Medical Journal.*

Brnighausen, T., *Medizinische Humanexperimente der japanischen Truppen für Biologische Kriegsfhrung in China, 1932–1945* (Diss. med., Med. Fak., Univ. Heidelberg, 1996).

Brodie, Janet Farrell, *Contraception and Abortion in 19th-century America* (Ithaca & London, 1994).

Brookes, Barbara, *Abortion in England 1900–1967* (London, 1988).

Brosig, W. & Nagel, R., *Nierentransplantation* (Berlin, 1965).

Brown, C.G., *The People in the Pews: Religion and Society in Scotland since 1780* (Dundee, 1993).

Brugger, Claudia Maria, *Zur Entwicklung des Obduktionswesens aus medizinischer und rechtlicher Sicht* (Thesis Med. Fak., Univ. Heidelberg, 1977).

Brugger, Claudia Maria & Kühn, Hermann, *Sektion der menschlichen Leiche. Zur Entwicklung des Obduktionswesens aus medizinischer und rechtlicher Sicht* (Stuttgart, 1979), 100–13.

BSHC Executive Committee, *Minutes*, CMAC, Wellcome Institue for the History of Medicine.

Büchner, Franz, 'Gedenkrede auf Ludwig Aschoff, gehalten bei der Gedenkfeier der Universität Freiburg am 5. Dezember 1943' (*Feldpostbrief der Medizinischen Fakultät der Universität Freiburg/Brsg.*, Nr.4) (Freiburg, 1943), 1–24.

Büchner, Franz, 'Ludwig Aschoff' in Vincke, Johannes (ed.), *Freiburger Professoren des 19. und 20. Jahrhunderts* (Freiburg i.Br., 1957), 11–20.

Buckley, S., 'The Failure to Resolve the Problem of Venereal Disease Among the Troops in Britain During World War I' in Bond, B. & Roy, I.(eds.), *War and Society. A Yearbook of Military History*, Vol. 2 (London, 1977), 65–85

Budd, Susan & Sharma, Ursula (eds.), *The Healing Bond. The patient–practitioner relationship and therapeutic responsibility* (London & New York, 1994).

Buhl, Ludwig, *Ueber die Stellung und Bedeutung der pathologischen Anatomie* (München, 1863).

Burke, E.T., *The Venereal Problem* (London, 1919).

Burke, E.T., 'Are we to have Compulsory Treatment of Venereal Disease?', *Health & Empire*, New Series 10 (1935), 120–23.

Buscher, Dorothea, *Die wissenschaftstheoretischen, medizinhistorischen und zeitkritischen Arbeiten von Ludwig Aschoff* (Thesis, Med. Fac., Freiburg i.Br., 1980).

Bushe, K.-A. (ed.), *Fortschritte auf dem Gebiet der Neurochirurgie* (Stuttgart, 1970).

Bynum, W.F., 'Reflections on the History of Human Experimentation' in. Spicker, S.F. et al. (eds.), *The Use of Human Beings in Research with Special Reference to Clinical Trials* (Dordrecht, Boston & London, 1988), 29–46.

Bynum, W.F. & Porter, Roy (eds.), *William Hunter and the Eighteenth-Century Medical World* (Cambridge, 1985).

Bynum, W.F. & Porter Roy (eds.), *Medical Fringe and Medical Orthodoxy 1750–1850* (London, Sydney, Wolfeboro, 1987).

Bynum, W.F. & Porter, Roy (eds.), *Companion Encyclopedia of the History of Medicine*, 2 Vols. (London & New York, 1993).

Byrne, P. (ed.), *Health, Rights and Resources* (London, 1988).


Caro Baroja, *Los judíos*, Vol. 3, 55–131.

Charcot, J.M. & Magnan, V., 'Inversion du sens génital', *Archive de neurologie*, 3–4 (1882), 53–60, 296–322.

Chevalier, Julian, *Sur l'inversion de l'instinct sexuel au point de vue médico-légal* (Lyon, 1893).

Chisholm, J. (ed.), *Green's Encyclopaedia of the Law of Scotland* (Edinburgh, 1911).

Church of Scotland, *Reports to General Assembly* (1944).

Clark, A.J., *Applied Pharmacology* (London, 1937).

Clark, M. & Crawford, C. (eds.), *Legal Medicine in History* (Cambridge, 1994).

Comte, August, *System of Positive Polity* (London, 1877).

Contreras, Jaime, *Sotos contra Riquelmes. Regidores, inquisidores y criptojudíos* (Madrid, 1992).

Contreras, Jaime, 'Las modificaciones estructurales. Los cambios en la Península' in *Historia de la Inquisición en España y América*, Vol. 1, 1156–77.

Cooter, R. (ed.), *Studies in the History of Alternative Medicine* (Oxford, 1988).

Cooter, R., 'The Resistible Rise of Medical Ethics', *Social History of Medicine*, 8 (1995), 257–70.

Corbin, A., *Women for Hire: Prostitution and Sexuality in France after 1850* (Cambridge MA & London, 1990).

Corson, J.F., 'Sleeping Sickness in the Ikoma District of Tanganyika Territory: Notes on Some Cases Treated by Professor F.K. Kleine', *Annals of Tropical Medicine and Parasitology*, 22 (1928), 379–418.

Corson, J.F., 'A record of some complications which occurred in the course of experimental infections of African volunteers with *Trypanosoma rhodesiense*', *Annals of Tropical Medicine and Parasitology*, 32 (1938), 437–43.

Cox-Maksimov, D., *The Making of the Clinical Trial in Britian, 1910–1945: Expertise, the State and the Public* (PhD thesis, University of Cambridge, 1997).

Credé, Carl, *Paragraph 218, Gequälte Menschen* (Tortured people).

Cuenca, Archivo Diocesano, *Inquisición*.

Culmann, H.-M., *Zur geschichtlichen Entwicklung der Todesauffassung des Arztes im europäischen Raum* (Diss. med., Freiburg i. Brei., 1986).

Cunningham, George J., *The History of British Pathology* (Bristol, 1993).

Currer, Caroline & Stacey, Margaret (eds.), *Concepts of Health, Illness and Disease. Comparative Perspective* (Providence & Oxford, 1986).

Cushney, A.R., *A Textbook of Pharmacology and Therapeutics: Or the Action of Drugs in Health and Disease* (London, 1910).


d'Almeras, H., *Le Marquis de Sade* (Paris, 1906).

*Dagblad voor Noord-Limburg*.

Dallemagne, Jules, *Théories de la criminalité* (Paris, 1896).

Darnton, Robert. *The Great Cat Massacre and Other Episodes in French Cultural History* (New York, 1984).

Davidson, R., '"A Scourge to be firmly gripped": The Campaign for VD Controls in Interwar Scotland', *Social History of Medicine*, 6 (1993), 213–35.

Davidson, R., 'Venereal Disease, Sexual Morality, and Public Health in Interwar Scotland', *Journal of the History of Sexuality*, 5 (1994), 267–94.

Davidson, R., 'Fighting "the Deadly Scourge": The Impact of World War II on Civilian VD policy in Scotland', *Scottish Historical Review*, 75 (1996), 72–97.

Davis, Natalie Zemon, *Fiction in the Archives. Pardon Tales and their Tellers in Sixteenth-Century France* (Stanford CA, 1987).

*De Amsterdammer*.

*De Grondwet*.

*de Maasbode*.

Debate in the House of Commons on the Criminal Law Amendment Bill, *Hansard*, [HC] 90, 19 Feb. 1917, cols. 1098–131

Dedieu, Jean Pierre, 'Le quatre temps de l'Inquisition' in Bennassar, B. et al., *L'Inquisition espagnole XVe–XIXe siècle* (Paris, 1979), pp. 16–41

*Der Spiegel*

Deutscher Textilarbeiterverband (ed.), *Mein Arbeitstag, mein Wochenende. 150 Berichte von Textilarbeiterinnen* (Berlin, 1930).

Deutsches Hygiene Museum, Dresden (ed.), *Unter anderen Umständen. Zur Geschichte der Abtreibung* (Berlin, 1993).

Díaz, Galende, *La crisis del siglo XVIII y la Inquisición española. El caso de la Inquisición toledana (1700–1820)* (Madrid, 1988)

*Die Welt.*

*Die Zeit.*

Dienel, Christiane, 'Das 20. Jahrhundert (I). Frauenbewegung, Klassenjustiz und das Recht auf Selbstbestimmung der Frau' in Jütte, Robert (ed.), *Geschichte der Abtreibung. Von der Antike bis zur Gegenwart* (Munich, 1993).

Dinges, M. (ed.), *Medizinkritische Bewegungen im Deutschen Reich (ca. 1870–ca. 1933)* (Stuttgart, 1996).

Dinges, M. & Schlich, T.(eds), *Neue Wege in der Seuchengeschichte* (Stuttgart, 1995).

Doerr, Wilhelm, 'Geleitwort' in Brugger, Claudia Maria & Kühn, Hermann, *Sektion der menschlichen Leiche. Zur Entwicklung des Obduktionswesens aus medizinischer und rechtlicher Sicht* (Stuttgart, 1979).

Domínguez Ortiz, Antonio & Vincent, Bernard, *Historia de los moriscos. Vida y tragedia de una minoría* (Madrid, 1985).

*Dordrechts Nieuwsblad.*

Dowbiggin, Ian R., *Inheriting Madness: Professionalization and Psychiatric Knowledge in Nineteenth-Century France* (Berkeley, 1991).

Duden, Barbara, *The Woman beneath the Skin* (Cambridge MA, 1991).

Dumont, Arsène, *Dépopulation et civilisation: étude démographique* (Béjin, André (ed.) (Paris, 1990)), 402–10.


Eckart, W.U., 'The Colony as laboratory and the fight against sleeping sickness in German East Africa and Togo' (forthcoming).

Eckart, Wolfgang U. & Gradmann, Christoph (eds.), *Ärzte-Lexikon. Von der Antike bis zum 20. Jahrhundert* (München, 1995).

Eckart, Wolfgang U. & Gradmann, Christoph (eds.), *Die Medizin und der Erste Weltkrieg* (Neuere Medizin- und Wissenschaftsgeschichte. Quellen und Studien, Vol. 3) (Pfaffenweiler, 1996)

Eder, Franz, Hall, Lesley & Hekma, Gert (eds.), *Sexual Cultures in Europe* (Manchester, 1999).

Egido, Teófanes, 'La Inquisición en la España borbónica: el declive del Santo Oficio y la nueva coyuntura' in *Historia de la Inquisición en España y América*, Vol. 1, 1204–11.

Eisenmenger, W., Betz, P. & Penning, R., 'Arztrechtliche Fragen in der Pathologie I. Zur Rechtslage bei klinischen Sektionen', *Der Pathologe*, 12 (1991), 126–30.

*Eleventh Annual Report of the Ministry of Health, P.P. 1930–31* (Cmd.3667) XIII.

Elkeles, B., 'Medizinische Menschenversuche gegen Ende des 19. Jahrhunderts und der Fall Neisser. Rechtfertigung und Kritik einer wissenschaftlichen Methode', *Medizinhistorisches Journal*, 20 (1985), 135–48.

Ellenberger, H. F., *The Discovery of the Unconscious* (New York, 1970).

Ellis, Havelock, *Studies in the Psychology of Sex* (New York, 1936).

Emergency Powers (Defence) General Regulations, 5 November 1942, *Statutory Rules and Orders* (1942), Vol. 2, 89–94.

Emmrich, M., 'Hirntod und Organtransplantation. Debatte im Bundestag über das neue Organtransplantationsgesetz', *Dr. med. Mabuse*, 106, März/April (1997), 22–24.

Enactment of the Prussian War Ministry, 14 July 1915, and of the Bavarian War Ministry, 19 August 1915, Bayerisches Hauptstaatsarchiv, IV, MKr10103.

Engelhardt, Dietrich v. & Hartmann, Fritz (eds.), *Klassiker der Medizin*, 2 vols (Munich, 1991).

Engelhardt, Dietrich v., 'Romantische Mediziner' in Engelhardt, Dietrich v. & Hartmann, Fritz (eds.), *Klassiker der Medizin*, Vol. 2 (Munich, 1991), 95–118.

Engisch, K., 'Über Rechtsfragen bei homologer Organtransplantation. Ergänzende Bemerkungen aus der Sicht des Juristen (des Kriminalisten)', *Der Chirurg*, 38 (1967), 252–55.

*Entscheidungen des Reichsgerichts in Strafsachen.*

Escudero, J. A., *Perfiles jurídicos de la Inquisición española* (Madrid, 1989).

*Estate Ludwig Aschoff, div. V/2. Vor und im Ersten Weltkrieg*, Institut für Geschichte der Medizin, Freiburg i.Br.

Eulner, Hans-Heinz, *Die Entwicklung der medizinischen Spezialfächer an den Universitäten des deutschen Sprachgebietes* (Stuttgart, 1970).

Evans, D., 'Tackling the "Hideous Scourge": The Creation of the Venereal Disease Treatment Centres in Early Twentieth-Century Britain', *Social History of Medicine*, 5 (1992), 413–33.

Evans, R.J., *Death in Hamburg: Society and Politics in the Cholera-Years 1830–1910* (Oxford, 1987).

Eyler, J.M., *Sir Arthur Newsholme and State Medicine, 1885–1935* (Cambridge, 1997).


Faden, R.& Beauchamp, T., *A History and Theory of Informed Consent* (New York, 1986).

Faulder, C., *Whose Body Is It? The Troubling Issue of Informed Consent* (London, 1985).

Feigl, W. & Leitner, H., 'Die hohe Autopsierate Österreichs und ihre Gründe', *Der Pathologe*, 7 (1986), 4–7.

Féré, Charles, *Pathologie des émotions* (Paris, 1892).

*Festgabe für Richard Schmidt. Zu seinem siebzigsten Geburtstag am 19. Januar 1932 überreicht von Verehrern und Schülern* (Leipzig, 1932).

*Final Report of the Royal Commission on Venereal Diseases*, P.P. 1916 (Cd. 8189) XVI.

Fischer, A., *Geschichte des deutschen Gesundheitswesens*, Vol. 2 (Berlin, 1933).

Fischer, Walther, 'Ludwig Aschoff. 1866–1942' in Freund, Hugo & Berg, Alexander (eds.), *Geschichte der Mikroskopie. Leben und Werk grosser Forscher*, Vol. 2 (Frankfurt/M., 1964), 13–21.

Fischer, Walther & Gruber, Georg B., *Fünfzig Jahre Pathologie in Deutschland* (Stuttgart, 1949).

Fischer-Homberger, Esther, *Medizin vor Gericht: Gerichtsmedizin von der Renaissance bis zur Aufklärung* (Bern, 1983).

Fleming, P.J., 'Fighting the "Red Plague": Observations on the Response to Venereal Disease in New Zealand 1910–45', *New Zealand Journal of History*, 22 (1988), 56–64.

Forgan, R., 'Compulsory Treatment of Venereal Diseases', *Medical Officer*, 39 (1928), 269–71.

Fortuyn, H.J.W., Drooglever, *Kwakzalverij, bijgeloof en geneeskunst* (Amsterdam, 1940).

Foster, William Derek, *A Short History of Clinical Pathology* (Edinburgh & London, 1961).

Foster, William Derek, *Pathology as a profession in Great Britain and the early history of the Royal College of Pathologists* (London, 1983).

Fourquet, Émile, *Vacher* (Paris, 1931).

Fox, R.C. (ed.), *Essays in Medical Sociology. Journeys into the Field* (New York, 1979).

Fox, R.C. & Swazey, J.P., *The Courage to Fail. A Social View of Organ Transplants and Dialysis* (Chicago & London, 1974).

*Frankfurter Allgemeine Zeitung.*

Franzblau, M.J., 'Ethical Values in Health Care in 1995: Lessons from the Nazi Period', *Journal of the Medical Association of Georgia*, 84 (1995), 161–64.

Fraser, P., *Treatise on Husband and Wife According to the Law of Scotland*, Vol. 2, 2nd edition (Edinburgh, 1878).

Freund, Hugo & Berg, Alexander (eds.), *Geschichte der Mikroskopie. Leben und Werk grosser Forscher* (Frankfurt/M., 1964).

Frewer, A., Köhler, M. & Rödel, C. (eds.), *Herztransplantation und Ethik. Historische und philosophische Aspekte eines paradigmatischen Eingriffs der modernen Medizin* (Erlangen, Jena (Erlanger Studien zur Ethik in der Medizin, Bd. 4), 1996.

Frowein, R.A., Euler, K.H. & Karim-Nejad, A., 'Grenzen der Wiederbelebung bei schweren Hirntraumen', *Langenbecks Archiv für klinische Chirurgie*, 308 (1964), 276–81.

Gallwas, H.-U., Geilen, G., Geisler L., et al., 'Wissenschaftler für ein tragfähiges Transplantationsgesetz', *Zeitschrift für Allgemeinmedizin*, 71 (1995), 1109–12.

Gänshirt, H., Berlit, P. & Haack, G. (eds.), *Kardiovaskuläre Erkrankungen und Nervensystem, Neurotoxikologie, Probleme des Hirntodes* (Berlin & Heidelberg, 1985).

García Ballester, Luis, 'The minority of Morisco Physicians in the Spain of the 16th Century and their Conflicts in a Dominant Christian Society', *Sudhoffs Archiv*, 60 (1976), 209–34

García Ballester, Luis, *Los moriscos y la medicina* (Barcelona, 1984).

García Ballester, Luis, 'Academicism versus empiricism in practical medicine in sixteenth-century Spain with regard to Morisco practitioners' in Wear, A., French, R.K. & Lonie, I.M. (eds.), *The medical renaissance of the sixteenth-century* (Cambridge, 1985), 246–70.

García Ballester, Luis, 'Medical Ethics in Transition in the Latin Medicine of the Thirteenth and Fourteenth Centuries: New Perspectives on the Physician–Patient Relationship and the Doctor's fee' in Wear, A., Geyer-Kordesch, J. & French, R. (eds.), *Doctors and Ethics: The Earlier Historical Setting of Professional Ethics* (Amsterdam & Atlanta, 1993), 38–71.

García Ballester, Luis, 'The Inquisition and minority medical practitioners in Counter-Reformation Spain' in Grell, O.P. & Cunningham, A. (eds.), *Medicine and the Reformation* (London & New York, 1993), 156–91.

García Ballester, Luis, 'Ethical problems in the relationship between doctors and patients in fourteenth-century Spain: on Christian and Jewish practitioners' in Kottek, Samuel S. & García Ballester, Luis (eds.), *Medicine and Medical Ethics in Medieval and Early Modern Spain* (Jerusalem, 1996), 11–32.

García Ballester, Luis, 'Minorities and Medicine in Sixteenth-Century Spain: Judaizers, "Moriscos" and the Inquisition' in Kottek, Samuel S. & García Ballester, Luis (eds.), *Medicine and Medical Ethics in Medieval and Early Modern Spain* (Jerusalem, 1996), 119–35.

Garcia Cárcel, Ricardo, 'El funcionamiento estructural de la Inquisición inicial' in *Historia de la Inquisición en España y América*, Vol. 1, 405–33.

García Cárcel, Ricardo, 'Ascens i decadència de la historiografia de la Inquisició', *L'Avenç*, no. 210 (January 1997), 18–23.

Garnier, Paul, 'Des Perversions sexuelles obsédantes et impulsives', *Archives de l'anthropologie criminelle*, 15 (1900), 618.

Garnier, Pierre, *Anomalies sexuelles: apparentes et cachées* (Paris, 1889).

Gärtner, A. (ed.), *Weyls Handbuch der Hygiene*, Vol. 8 (Leipzig, 2nd edition, 1918–22).

*Gazette de Tribunaux.*

Geiger, Paul, 'Leiche' in Hoffmann-Krayer, E. et al. (*Handwörterbuch zur deutschen Volkskunde, Abt.1: Aberglaube*), Vols. 1–10 (Berlin, 1927–42); Vol. VIII (Berlin/Leizig, 1936–37).

Geiger, Paul, 'Leichenschändung' in Bächtold-Stäubli, Hanns et al. (eds.), '*Handwörterbuch des Deutschen Aberglaubens*' (*Handwörterbuch zur deutschen Volkskunde, Abt.1: Aberglaube*), Vols. 1–10 (Berlin 1927–42), Vol. 5 (Berlin & Leipzig, 1932–33), col. 1093–94.

Geiger, Paul, 'Tote (der)' in Bächtold-Stäubli, Hanns et al. (eds.), '*Handwörterbuch des Deutschen Aberglaubens*' (*Handwörterbuch zur deutschen Volkskunde, Abt.1: Aberglaube*), Vols. 1–10 (Berlin, 1927–42). Vol. 8 (Berlin & Leipzig, 1936–37), col. 1019–34.

Geilen, G., 'Das Leben des Menschen in den Grenzen des Rechts. Zu den Wandlungen des Todesbegriffs und zu neuen Schutzproblemen des werdenden Lebens', *Zeitschrift für das gesamte Familienrecht*, 15 (1968), 121–30.

Geilen, G., 'Medizinischer Fortschritt und juristischer Todesbegriff' in Lüttger, H., Blei, H & Hanau, P. (eds.), *Festschrift für Ernst Heinitz zum 70. Geburtstag* (Berlin, 1972), 373–96.

Geilen, G., 'Rechtsfragen der Organtransplantation' in Honecker, M. (ed.), *Aspekte und Probleme der Organtransplantation* (Neukirchen-Vluyn, 1973), 179.

Geilen, G., 'Rechtsfragen der Todeszeitbestimmung' in Krösl, W. & Scherzer E. (eds.), *Die Bestimmung des Todeszeitpunktes. Kongreß in der Wiener Hofburg vom 4. bis 6. Mai 1972* (Wien, 1973), 285–93.

Geison, Gerald L. (ed.), *Professions and the French State* (Philadelphia, 1984).

Gelfand, Toby, *Professionalizing Modern Medicine. Paris Surgeons and Medical Science and Institutions in the 18th Century* (Westport CT, 1980).

Gelfand, Toby, 'The History of the Medical Profession' in Bynum, W.F. & Porter, Roy (eds.), *Companion Encyclopedia of the History of Medicine*, Vol. 2 (London & New York, 1993), 1119–50.

Gerlach, J., 'Syndrome des Sterbens und der Vita reducta', *Münchener medizinische Wochenschrift*, 111 (1969), 169–76.

Gerlach, J., 'Gehirntod und totaler Tod', *Münchener medizinische Wochenschrift*, 111 (1969), 732–36.

Gerlach, J., 'Bedeutet Gehirntod auch menschlichen Tod?', *Fortschritte der Medizin*, 88 (1970), 399–400.

Gerrens, U., *Medizinisches Ethos und theologische Ethik. Karl und Dietrich Bonhoeffer in den Auseinandersetzungen um Zwangssterilisation und 'Euthanasie' im Nationalsozialismus* (Munich, 1996).

*Gesetz über die Spende, Entnahme und Übertragung von Organen* (Transplantationsgesetz-TPG), Bundestagsdrucksache 13/8027.

Giddens, A., 'Living in a Post-Traditional Society' in Beck, U., Giddens, A. & Lash, S. (eds.), *Reflexive Modernization. Politics, Tradition and Aesthetics in the Modern Social Order* (Cambridge, 1994), 56–109.

Gijswijt-Hofstra, Marijke (ed.), *Geloven in genezen* (Amsterdam, 1991).

Gijswijt-Hofstra, Marijke, 'Homeopathy's early Dutch conquests: the Rotterdam Clientele of Clemens von Bönninghausen in the 1840s and 1850s', *Journal of the History of Medicine and Allied Sciences* 51 (1996) 155–83.

Gijswijt-Hofstra, Marijke, Marland, Hilary & Witt, Hans de (eds.), *Illness and Healing Alternatives in Western Europe* (London, 1997).

Gley, E., 'Les Aberrations de l'instinct sexuel', *Revue philosophique*, 17 (1884), 66–92.

Glyn-Hughes, F., Lourie, E.M. & Yorke, W., 'Studies in Chemotherapy XVII: The Action of Undecane Diamidine in Malaria', *Annals of Tropical Medicine and Parasitology*, 32 (1938), 103–07.

Goldschmid, Edgar, *Entwicklung und Bibliographie der pathologisch-anatomischen Abbildung* (Leipzig, 1925).

Goldstein, Jan, *Console and Classify: The French Psychiatric Profession in the Nineteenth Century* (Cambridge, 1987).

Goldworth, A., 'Informed Consent in the Human Genome Enterprise', *Cambridge Quarterly of Healthcare Ethics*, 4 (1995), 296–303.

Good, B.J., *Medicine, rationality and experience* (Cambridge, 1994).

Göppinger, H. (ed.), *Arzt und Recht. Medizinisch-juristische Grenzprobleme unserer Zeit* (München, 1966).

Gordon, R.M., 'Emetine Periodide in the Treatment of *S. heamatobium* Infections Among West African Children', *Annals of Tropical Medicine and Parasitology*, 20 (1926), 229–37.

Gottlieb, M.S. et al., *Current Topics in AIDS* (Chichester, 1989).

Gray, B.H., *Human Subjects in Medical Experimentation: A Sociological Study of the Conduct and Regulation of Clinical Research* (New York, 1975).

Grell, O.P. & Cunningham, A. (eds.), *Medicine and the Reformation* (London & New York, 1993).

Grossmann, Anita, *Reforming Sex* (New York & Oxford, 1995).

Grossmann, Anita, 'Abortion and the Economic Crisis: The 1931 Campaign against Paragraph 218' in Bridenthal, Renate, Grossmann, Atina & Kaplan, Marion (eds.), *When Biology Became Destiny* (New York, 1984), 66–86.

Gründel, J., 'Der relative Wert irdisch leiblichen menschlichen Lebens und der Tod aus theologischer Perspektive' in Krösl, W. & Scherzer, E. (eds.), *Die Bestimmung des Todeszeitpunktes. Kongreß in der Wiener Hofburg vom 4. bis 6. Mai 1972* (Wien, 1973), 321–27.

Grynaeus, Tamás, 'Weiterleben der heilenden Volksbräuche und -glauben in einem neugesiedelten Dorf in Ungarn', *Curare*, 3 & 4 (1993), 191–92.

Guarnieri, Patrizia, *A Case of Child Murder: Law and Science in Nineteenth-Century Tuscany* (Cambridge, 1993).

Gütgemann, A. & Käufer, C., 'Organentnahme und Transplantation', *Deutsche medizinische Wochenschrift*, 96 (1971), 609–14.

Guttstadt, Albert (ed.), *Die naturwissenschaftlichen und medicinischen Staatsanstalten Berlins. Festschrift für die 59. Versammlung deutscher Naturforscher und Aerzte* (Berlin, 1886).


Haim, A. (ed.), *Society and Community* (Jerusalem, 1991).

Hamlin, C., 'State Medicine in Great Britain' in Porter, D. (ed.), *The History of Public Health and the Modern State* (Amsterdam, 1994), 132–64.

Hanack, E.-W., 'Todeszeitbestimmung, Reanimation und Organtransplantation', *Deutsches Ärzteblatt*, 66/19 (1969), 1320–31.

Hanack, E.-W., 'Rechtsprobleme bei Organtransplantationen', *Studium Generale*, 23 (1970), 428–43.

*Hansard.*

Harkness, J.M., 'Prisoners and Pellagra', *Public Health Reports*, 111 (1996), 463–67.

Harley, David, 'Political Post-mortems and Morbid Anatomy in Seventeenth-century England', *Social History of Medicine*, 7 (1994), 1–28.

Harris, Ruth, *Murders and Madness: Medicine, Law, and Society in the Fin-de-Siècle* (Oxford, 1989).

Harrison, L.W., 'Venereal Diseases' in MacNalty, A.S. (ed.), *The Civilian Health and Medical Services*, Vol. 1 (London, 1953), 120–01.

Harrison, L.W., Ward, D.C.L., Ferguson, T. & Rorke, Margaret, *Report on Anti-Venereal Measures in Certain Scandinavian Countries and Holland* (London, 1938).

Harrison, M. & Cooter, R. (eds.), *War, Medicine and Modernity, 1860–1945* (Stroud, 1999).

Haury, Dr., 'Les faux témoins pathologiques', *Archives de l'anthropologie criminelle*, 27 (1912), 637–53.

Haustein, H., 'The German Federal Law for Combatting Venereal Diseases', *Health & Empire*, New Series 2 (1927), 89–99.

Heckhausen, Christel, *Anatomen und Anatomie im Urteil der Öffentlichkeit seit 1500* (Berlin, Diss.Med.Fak., 1966).

Heinitz, E., *Rechtliche Fragen der Organtransplantation* (Berlin, 1970).

Helman, C.G., *Culture, Health and Illness* (4th ed.) (Oxford & Woburn MA, 2000).

Henningsen, Gustav, 'El banco de datos del Santo Oficio. Las relaciones de causas de la Inquisición española (1550–1700)', *Boletín de la Real Academia de la Historia*, 174 (1977), 547–70.

Henningsen, Gustav, *The Witches' advocate: basque witchcraft and the Spanish Inquisition, 1609–1614* (Reno, 1980).

Henningsen, Gustav, Tedeschi, John & Amiel, Charles (eds.), *The Inquisition in Early Modern Europe: Studies in Sources and Method* (Dekalb, Ill. 1984).

Henoch, Eduard, *Beiträge zur Kinderheilkunde* (Berlin, 1861).

Henry, Charles, *La Verité sur le marquis de Sade* (Paris, 1887).

Heuer, Stefanie & Conrads, Christoph, 'Aktueller Stand der Transplantationsgesetzgebung 1997', *Medizinrecht*, 5 (1997), 195–202.

Heym, Georg, 'Die Sektion' in Rölleke, Heinz (ed.), *Georg Heym Lesebuch: Gedichte, Prosa, Träume, Tagebücher* (Munich, 1984), 181–83.

Higonnet, M.R., et al. (eds.), *Behind the Lines: Gender and the Two World Wars* (New Haven, 1987).

*Historia de la Inquisición en España y América* (Madrid, 1984).

Hoff, J. & Schmitten, J. in der, 'Tot?', *Die Zeit*, No. 47 (1992), 56.

Hoff, J. & Schmitten, J. in der, 'Organspende – nur über meine Leiche?', *Die Zeit*, No. 7 (1993), 40.

Hoff, J. & Schmitten, J. in der (eds.), *Wann ist der Mensch tot? Organverpflanzung und Hirntodkriterium* (Reinbek, 1994).

Hoffmann-Krayer, E. et al. (*Handwörterbuch zur deutschen Volkskunde, Abt.1: Aberglaube*), Vols. 1–10 (Berlin, 1927–42).

Höfling, W. & Rixen, S., *Verfassungsfragen der Transplantationsmedizin* (Tübingen, 1996).

Hohlfeld, R. & Lau, C. (eds.), *Wissenschaft und reflexive Modernisierung* (Finck, 1998).

*Homenatge al Doctor Sebastià Garcia Martínez* (Valencia, 1988).

Honecker, M. (ed.), *Aspekte und Probleme der Organverpflanzung* (Neukirchen-Vluyn, 1973).

Honecker, M., 'Freiheit, den Tod anzunehmen. Theologische Gedanken aus Anlaß der Organtransplantationen' in Honecker, M. (ed.), *Aspekte und Probleme der Organverpflanzung* (Neukirchen-Vluyn, 1973), 183–203.

Hornblum, A.M., 'They Were Cheap and Available: Prisoners as Research Subjects in Twentieth Century America', *British Medical Journal*, 315 (ii) (1997), 1437–41.

Hort, Irmgard, *Die Pathologischen Institute der deutschsprachigen Universitäten (1850–1914)* (Thesis, Med. Fak., Köln, 1987)


Iserson, Kenneth V., *Death to Dust. What happens to dead Bodies?* (Tucson AZ, 1994).


Jackson, Margaret, *The 'Real' Facts of Life: Feminism and the Politics of Sexuality 1850–1940* (London, 1994).

Janzen, J.M., *The Quest for Therapy in Lower Zaire* (Berkeley, 1978).

Johnstone, R.W., *Report on Venereal Diseases*, Parliamentary Papers, 1913 (Cd.7029) XXXII.

Joly, Henri, *Le Crime: étude sociale* (Paris, 1888).

Jones, J.H., *Bad Blood: The Tuskegee Syphilis Experiment* (New York, 1993).

*Juristenzeitung.*

Jütte, Robert (ed.), *Geschichte der Abtreibung. Von der Antike bis zur Gegenwart* (Munich, 1993).

Jütte, Robert, Risse, Guenter B. & Woodward, John (eds.), *Culture, Knowledge and Healing: Historical Perspectives of Homeopathic Medicine in Europe and North America* (Sheffield, 1998).

Kaiser, G., 'Künstliche Insemination und Transplantation. Juristische und rechtspolitische Probleme' in Göppinger, H. (ed.), *Arzt und Recht. Medizinisch-juristische Grenzprobleme unserer Zeit* (München, 1966), 58–95.

Kaplan, Josef, 'The Portuguese Community of Amsterdam in the 17th Century. Between Tradition and Change' in Haim, A. (ed.), *Society and Community* (Jerusalem, 1991).

Katz, J., *The Silent World of Doctor and Patient* (New York & London, 1984).

Katz, O., 'Erst das Skalpell, dann die Moral', *Süddeutsche Zeitung*, No. 26, 30. Jan. 1968, 8.

Keun, Irmgard, *Gilgi – eine von uns* (Berlin, 1931).

Kirchheim, D. & Robertson, R.D., 'Biologische Grundlagen und Fortschritte in der Nierentransplantation. II. Patienten- und Spenderwahl, Organkonservierung', *Der Urologe*, 6 (1967), 67–74.

Klee, Ernst, *Auschwitz, die NS-Medizin und ihre Opfer* (Frankfurt/M., 1997).

Kleine, F.K., 'Report on the New Sleeping Sickness Focus at Ikoma', *Final Report of the League of Nations International Committee on Human Trypanosomiasis*, 1928.

Kleinman, A., 'Suffering in China and the West: The Challenge of an Interpersonal Locus of Experience to the Hypertrophy of Individual Autonomy in Health' in Woodward, John & Jütte, Robert (eds.), *Coping with Sickness. Perspectives on Health Care, Past and Present* (Sheffield, 1996) 43–52.

Klinkhammer, G., 'Diskussion um das Transplantationsgesetz. Wann ist der Mensch tot?', *Deutsches Ärzteblatt*, 94/10 (1997), (C) 430–32.

Kniesche, T.W. & Brockmann, S. (eds.), *Dancing on the Volcano. Essays on the Culture of the Weimar Republic* (Columbia, 1994).

Kohlhaas, M., 'Zur Feststellung des Todeszeitpunktes Verstorbener', *Deutsche medizinische Wochenschrift*, 93 (1968), 412–14.

Kommission für Reanimation und Organtransplantation der Deutschen Gesellschaft für Chirurgie, 'Todeszeichen und Todeszeitbestimmung', *Der Chirurg*, 39 (1968), 196–97. English translation in Largiadèr, F. (ed.), *Organ Transplantation* (Stuttgart, 1970), Appendix 3.

Kooijman, Henk, *Volksverhalen uit het grensgebied van Zuid-Holland, Utrecht, Gelderland en Noord-Brabant* (Amsterdam, 1988).

Kottek, Samuel S. & García Ballester, Luis (eds.), *Medicine and Medical Ethics in Medieval and Early Modern Spain* (Jerusalem, 1996).

Krafft-Ebing, Richard von, *Psychopathia Sexualis* (tr. Franklin S. Klaf) (New York, 1965).

Kress, H., *Ärztliche Fragen bei der Organtransplantation* (Berlin, 1970).

Krietsch, Peter, 'Zur Geschichte der Prosektur der Charité Berlin, 1. Gründung der Prosektur und Philipp Phoebus als erster Prosektor', *Zentralblatt für allgemeine Pathologie und pathologische Anatomie*, 136 (1990), 377–87.

Krietsch, Peter, 'Zur Geschichte der Prosektur der Charité Berlin, 2. Mitteilung. Robert Friedrich Froriep, Prosektor der Charité von 1833 bis 1864', *Zentralblatt für allgemeine Pathologie und pathologische Anatomie*, 136 (1990), 729–38.

Kronfeld, E.M., *Der Krieg im Aberglauben und Volksglauben. Kulturhistorische Beiträge* (München, 1917).

Krösl, W. & Scherzer E. (eds.), *Die Bestimmung des Todeszeitpunktes. Kongreß in der Wiener Hofburg vom 4. bis 6. Mai 1972* (Wien, 1973).

Krüger, Martina, 'Kinderfachabteilung Wiesengrund. Die Tötung behinderter Kinder in Wittenau' in Arbeitsgruppe zur Erforschung der Geschichte der Karl-Bonhoeffer-Nervenklinik, scientific adviser Aly, Götz (eds.) *Totgeschwiegen 1933–1945. Zur Geschichte der Wittenauer Heilstätten. Seit 1957 Karl-Bonhoeffer-Nervenklinik* (Berlin, 1989), 151–76.

Krumbhaar, Edwin B., *Pathology* (Clio Medica XIX) (New York, 1937, repr. 1962).

Kudlien, Fridolf, 'Antike Anatomie und menschlicher Leichnam', *Hermes*, 97 (1969), 78–94.


Laborde, M.J.V. et al., *Étude psycho-physiologique, médico-légal & anatomique sur Vacher* (Paris, 1900).

Lacassagne, Alexandre, 'Péderastie', *Dictionnaire encyclopédique des sciences médicales*, 2nd series (Paris, 1886), 22, 239–59.

Lacassagne, Alexandre, 'Vacher l'Éventreur', *Archives de l'anthropologie criminelle*, 13 (1898), 641.

Lacassagne, Alexandre, 'Le cerveau de Vacher', *Archives de l'anthropologie criminelle*, 14 (1899), 653–62.

Lacassagne, Alexandre, *Vacher l'Éventreur et les crimes sadiques* (Lyon, 1899).

Lachmund, Jens & Stolberg, Gunnar, *Patientenwelten. Krankheit und Medizin vom späten 18. bis zum frühen 20. Jahrhundert im Spiegel von Autobiographien* (Opladen, 1995).

Lammel, Hans-Uwe, *Nosologische und therapeutische Konzeptionen in der romantischen Medizin* (Abhandlungen zur Geschichte der Medizin und der Naturwissenschaften, Vol. 59) (Husum, 1990).

Lamoureux, André, *De l'éventration au point de vue médico-légal* (Lyon, 1891).

Langan, M. & Schwarz, B. (eds.), *Crises in the British State, 1880–1930* (London, 1985).

Largiadèr, F. (ed.), *Organ Transplantation* (Stuttgart, 1970).

Largiadèr, F., 'History of Organ Transplantation' in Largiadèr, F. (ed.), *Organ Transplantation* (Stuttgart, 1970), 2–12.

Laufs, A., 'Juristische Probleme des Hirntodes' in Gänshirt, H., Berlit, P. & Haack, G. (eds.), *Kardiovaskuläre Erkrankungen und Nervensystem, Neurotoxikologie, Probleme des Hirntodes* (Berlin, Heidelberg, 1985), 559–64.

Laurent, Émile, *L'Anthropologie criminelle et les nouvelles théories du crime* (Paris, 1893).

Laurent, Émile, *La poésie décadente devant la science psychiatrique* (Paris, 1897).

Laurent, Émile, *Sadisme et masochisme* (Paris, 1903).

Laurent-Martin, M., *Le Roi des assassins* (Paris, 1897).

Laves, W., 'Agonie', *Münchener medizinische Wochenschrift*, 107 (1965), 113–18.

*Le Grand Robert de la langue française* (Paris, 1985).

Lea, Henry C., *The Moriscos of Spain. The Conversion and Expulsion* (London, 1901).

Lea, Henry C., *A History of the Inquisition of Spain*, 4 Vols. (New York, 1906–07).

Leavitt, J.W. & Numbers, R.L., *Sickness and Health in America* (Madison & London, 1985).

Lenz, Max, 'Sonderbarer Leichenkult in der Charité. Obduktion trotz Einspruchs der Hinterbliebenen. "Klinisches Interesse geht vor."', *Neue Berliner Zeitung*, No. 274 11th Vol., November 22, 1929.

Lera, Rafael de, 'La última gran persecución contra el judaísmo. El tribunal de Cuenca, 1718–1725' in Escudero, J.A., *Perfiles jurídicos de la Inquisición española* (Madrid, 1989), 805–37.

Liebhardt, E.W., 'Zivilrechtliche Probleme an der Grenze zwischen Leben und Tod', *Deutsche Zeitschrift für die gesamte gerichtliche Medizin*, 57 (1966), 31–36.

Liebhardt, E.W. & Wuermeling, H.-B., 'Juristische und medizinisch-naturwissenschaftliche Begriffsbildung und die Feststellung des Todeszeitpunktes', *Münchener medizinische Wochenschrift*, 110 (1968), 1661–65.

*Limburger Koerier.*

Lindemann, Mary, *Health & Healing in Eighteenth-Century Germany* (Baltimore & London, 1996).

Linke, D.B., 'Die dritte kopernikanische Wende. Transplantationsmedizin und personale Identität', *Ethica*, 1 (1993), 53–64.

Liszt, F.v., 'Der strafrechtliche Schutz gegen Gesundheitsgefährdung durch Geschlechtskranke Gutachten', *Zeitschrift für Bekämpfung der Geschlechtskrankheiten*, 1 (1903), 1–25.

Llorente, Juan A., *Histoire critique de l'Inquisition d'Espagne*, 4 Vols. (Paris, 1817–18).

Local Government Board, *Venereal Diseases Circulars* (London, 1916).

Local Government Board for Scotland, *Venereal Diseases Circulars* (Edinburgh, 1916).

Löffler, Peter, *Studien zum Totenbrauchtum in den Gilden, Bruderschaften und Nachbarschaften Westfalens vom Ende des 15. bis zum Ende des 19. Jahrhunderts* (Forschungen zur Volkskunde, Vol. 47) (Münster, 1975), 58–74.

Löhrs, Udo, 'Ethik in der Pathologie – Anmerkungen' in Engelhardt, Dietrich von. (ed.), *Ethik im Alltag der Medizin. Spektrum der Disziplinen zwischen Forschung und Therapie* (Basel, Boston & Berlin, 1997), 61–74.

Lombroso, Cesare, *L'Homme criminel* (Paris, 1887).

Long, Esmond R., *A History of American Pathology* (Springfield, 1962).

Long, Esmond R., *A History of Pathology* (Baltimore, 1928; New York, 1965).

López Piñero, José Mª., *Ciencia y técnica en la sociedad española de los siglos XVI y XVII* (Barcelona, 1979), 387–433.

López Piñero, José Mª. et al., *Bibliographia Medica Hispanica*, Vols. 1 (1475–1600) & 2 (1601–1700) (Valencia, 1987–89).

Lubarsch, Otto, *Ein bewegtes Gelehrtenleben. Erinnerungen und Erlebnisse. Kämpfe und Gedanken* (Berlin, 1931).

Lüttger, H., Blei, H & Hanau, P. (eds.), *Festschrift für Ernst Heinitz zum 70. Geburtstag* (Berlin, 1972).

Lyons, M., 'Death camps in the Congo: Administrative responses to Sleeping Sickness, 1903–1911', *Bulletin Society Social History of Medicine*, 34 (1984), 28–31.

*Maandblad tegen de kwakzalverij.*

MacDonald, Arthur, *Le Criminel-type dans quelque formes graves de la criminalité* (tr. Henry Coutagne) (Lyon, 1894).

Macfie, J.W. & Fraser, M.W., 'Oral Administration of Quinine or Quinine and Arsenic for Short Periods to Young Native Children Infected with Malignant Tertian Malaria', *Annals of Tropical Medicine and Parasitology*, 14 (1920–21), 83–91.

Macfie, J.W.S., 'Oral Administration of Quinine Sulphate Grains 20 to Adult Natives Infected with Malignant Tertian Malaria', *Annals of Tropical Medicine and Parasitology*, 14 (1920–21), 93–94.

Macfie, J.W.S., 'Oral Administration of Quinine Sulphate Grains 10 Daily for 2 Consecutive Days Only for Native School-boys Infected with Malignant Tertian Malaria', *Annals of Tropical Medicine and Parasitology*, 14 (1920–21), 95–109.

Maclean, G. & Fairburn, H., 'Treatment of Rhodesian Sleeping Sickness with Bayer 205 and Tryparasimide: Observations on 719 Cases', *Annals of Tropical Medicine and Parasitology*, 26 (1932), 157–89.

Macleod, R.M., 'Law, Medicine and Public Opinion: The Resistance to Compulsory Health Legislation 1870–1907', *Public Law* (1967), 107–28, 189–211.

MacNalty, A.S. (ed.), *The Civilian Health and Medical Services*, Vol. 1 (London, 1953).

Madrid, Archivo Histórico Nacional, *Inquisición*.

Maehle, Andreas-Holger, 'Einstellungen zur Sektion der menschlichen Leiche im 17. und 18. Jahrhundert', *Niedersächsisches Ärzteblatt*, 17 (1991), 1–5.

Mahood, L., *The Magdalenes: Prostitution in the Nineteenth Century* (London & New York, 1990).

Malan, M., '"Herrgott, es schlägt wieder". Die Herzverpflanzungen des Professor Barnard', *Der Spiegel*, No. 13 (1968), 109–22.

Marciat, 'Le Marquis de Sade et le sadisme' in Lacassagne, Alexandre, *Vacher l'Éventreur et les crimes sadiques* (Lyon, 1899), 185–238.

Martindale, W.H., *The Extra Pharmacopoeia* (London, 1915).

Martindale, W.H, 'A Note on Emetine Preparation for Rectal and Oral Use', *Transactions of the Royal Society of Tropical Medicine and Hygiene*, XVII (1923), 27–32.

Martínez Vidal, Alvar & Pardo Tomás, José, 'In tenebris adhuc versantes. La respuesta de los novatores españoles a la invectiva de Pierre Régis', *Dynamis*, 15 (1995), 301–40.

Mauge, Annelise, *L'Identité masculine en crise au tournant du siècle, 1871–1914* (Paris, 1987).

Maulitz, Russel C., *Morbid Appearances. The anatomy of pathology in the early nineteenth century* (Cambridge, 1987).

Maulitz, Russel C., 'The Pathological Tradition' in Bynum, William F. & Porter, Roy (eds.), *Companion Encyclopedia of the History of Medicine*, 2 Vols. (London & New York, 1993), Vol. 1, 169–91.

May, O., *The Prevention of Venereal Disease* (Oxford, 1918).

McCarthy, C.R., 'Historical Background of Clinical Trials Involving Women and Minorities', *Academic Medicine*, 69 (1994), 695–701.

McHugh, P., *Prostitution and Victorian Social Reform* (New York, 1980).

McLaren, Angus, *Birth Control in nineteenth-century England* (New York, 1978).

McLaren, Angus, *Trials of Masculinity: Policing Sexual Boundaries, 1870–1930* (Chicago, 1997 & 1999)

McNeill, P.M., *The Ethics and Politics of Human Experimentation* (Cambridge, 1993).

Méchoulan, Henry (ed.), *Les juifs d'Espagne. Histoire d'une diaspora, 1492–1992* (Paris, 1992).

Medick, Hans & Sabean, David Warren (eds.), *Interest and emotion. Essays on the study of family and kinship* (Cambridge, 1984).

Mehrhoff, F. & Müller, K.M., 'Klinische Sektion: erlaubt, notwendig, verboten?', *Der Pathologe*, 11 (1990), 131–36.

Meinel C. (ed.), *Instrument – Experiment* (Berlin, 2000).

Meseguer, Juan, 'Las primeras estructuras del Santo Oficio' in *Historia de la Inquisición en España y América* (Madrid, 1984), Vol. 1, 370–405.

Meeßen, Rudolf, *Die Freiburger Pathologie, ihre Entstehung und Fortentwicklung* (Thesis, Med. Fac., Freiburg i. Br., 1975).

Meyer, G.S., 'Criminal Punishment for the Transmission of Sexually Transmitted Diseases: Lessons from Syphilis', *Bulletin of the History of Medicine and Allied Sciences*, 65 (1991), 549–64.

Ministry of Health, *Sixth Annual Report of the Ministry of Health*, P.P. 1924–25 (Cmd.2724) XI.

Ministry of Health, 'Circular No 1956', 26 Jan. 1940, in *Medical Officer*, 63 (1940), 42–43.

Moll, Albert, *Die Konträre Sexualempfindung* (Berlin, 1893).

Mollaret, P. & Goulon, M. 'Le coma dépassé (mémoire préliminaire)', *Revue neurologique*, 101/1 (1959), 3–15.

Mollaret, P., 'Über die äußersten Möglichkeiten der Wiederbelebung. Die Grenzen zwischen Leben und Tod', *Münchener medizinische Wochenschrift*, 104 (1962), 1539–45.

Monter, William, *Frontiers of Heresy. The Spanish Inquisition from Basque Lands to Sicily* (Cambridge, 1990).

Mooij, A., *Out of Otherness: Characters and Narrators in the Dutch Venereal Disease Debates, 1850–1990* (Amsterdam & Atlanta, forthcoming).

Moore, F.D., *Transplantation. Geschichte und Entwicklung bis zur heutigen Zeit* (Engl. Original Philadelphia, London 1963) (Übersetzung aus dem Englischen mit einem Anhang von W. Brendel), (Berlin & Heidelberg, 1970).

Mörike, Klaus D., *Geschichte der Tübinger Anatomie* (Tübingen, 1988).

Muhs, R., Paulmann, J. & Steinmetz, W. (eds.), *Aneignung und Abwehr. Interkultureller Transfer zwischen Deutschland und Großbritannien im 19. Jahrhundert* (Bodenheim, forthcoming).

Murnane, M. & Daniels, K., 'Prostitutes as "Purveyors of Disease": Venereal Disease Legislation in Tasmania 1868–1945', *Hecate*, 5 (1979), 5–21.

NCCVD Executive Committee, *Minutes* (CMAC), Wellcome Institute for the History of Medicine.

*Nederlandsch tijdschrift voor geneeskunde.*

Neisser, A., *Die Geschlechtskrankheiten und ihre Bekämpfung. Vorschläge und Forderungen für Ärzte und Soziologen* (Berlin, 1916).

Netanyahu, B., *The Marranos of Spain Late 14th to Early 16th Century According to Contemporary Hebrew Sources* (New York, 1973).

Newman, George, 'The Present Position of Government Action in Venereal Disease' in *Proceedings of the Imperial Social Hygiene Congress at the British Empire Exhibition, May 12th–16th, 1924* (London, 1924), 19–21.

Newsholme, Arthur, 'Introduction' to Johnstone, R.W., *Report on Venereal Diseases*, *Parliamentary Papers, 1913* (Cd.7029) *XXXII.*

*Nieuwe Bredasche Courant.*

*Nieuwe Rotterdamsche Courant.*

*Nieuws van den Dag.*

*Noord Brabante.*

Nye, Robert, 'Heredity or Milieu: The Foundations of Modern European Criminological Theory', *Isis*, 67 (1976).

Nye, Robert, *Crime, Madness and Politics in Modern France: The Medical Concept of National Decline* (Princeton, 1984).

Nye, Robert, *Masculinity and Male Codes of Honor in Modern France* (New York, 1993).

Oberhoff, Günther, *Über die Rechtswidrigkeit und Strafbarkeit klinischer Leichensektionen* (Thesis Fac. Law Erlangen) (Emsdetten, 1935).

Ogawa, Teizo (ed.), *History of Pathology. Proceedings of the 8th international Symposium on the comparative history of Medicine – East and West (18–24 Sept. 1983, Susono-shi, Shizuoka, Japan)* (Tokyo, 1983).

Orth, Johannes, Das Pathologische Institut zu Berlin, *Berliner Klinische Wochenschrift*, 43 (1906), 817–26.

Osler, William, Science and Immortality (Boston, 1904).

Palacio Atard, V. et al., *La época de los primeros borbones I. La nueva monarquía y su posición en Europa (1700–1759)* (Madrid, 1987).

Pantel, Johannes & Bauer, Axel, 'Die Institutionalisierung der Pathologischen Anatomie im 19. Jahrhundert an den Universitäten Deutschlands, der deutschen Schweiz und Österreichs', *Gesnerus*, 47 (1990), 303–28.

Pappworth, M.H., *Human Guinea Pigs: Experimentation on Man* (London, 1967).

Pardo Tomás, José, 'Llorenç Coçar y la Inquisición valenciana', in *Homenatge al Doctor Sebastià Garcia Martínez* (Valencia, 1988), Vol. 1, 363–73.

Pardo Tomás, José & Martínez Vidal, Alvar, 'El Tribunal del Protomedicato y los médicos reales (1665–1724): entre la gracia real y la carrera profesional', *Dynamis*, 16 (1996), 59–89.

Paul, N. & Schlich, T. (eds.), *Medizingeschichte: Aufgaben, Probleme, Perspektiven* (Frankfurt/M. & New York, 1998).

Paul, Serge, *Le Vice et l'amour* (Paris, 1905).

Peiffer, Jürgen, *Hirnforschung im Zwielicht: Beispiele verführbarer Wissenschaft aus der Zeit des Nationalsozialismus. Julius Hallervorden – H.J. Scherer – Berthold Ostertag* (Abhandlungen zur Geschichte der Medizin und der Naturwissenschaften, Vol. 79) (Husum, 1997), 72–96.

Penin, H. & Käufer C. (eds.), *Der Hirntod. Todeszeitbestimmung bei irreversiblem Funktionsverlust des Gehirns* (Stuttgart, 1969).

Pérez Villanueva, Joaquín (ed.), *La Inquisición española. Nueva visión, nuevos horizontes* (Madrid, 1980).

Pernick, M.S., 'Back From the Grave: Recurring Controversies Over Defining and Diagnosing Death in History' in Zaner, R.M. (ed.), *Death: Beyond Whole-brain Criteria* (Dordrecht, 1988), 17–74.

Perrot, Michèle, 'The New Eve and the Old Adam; Changes in French Women's Condition at the Turn of the Century' in Higonnet, M.R. et al. (eds.), *Behind the Lines: Gender and the Two World Wars* (New Haven, 1987), 51–60.

Peukert, Detlev J.K., *The Weimar Republic. The Crisis of Classical Modernity* (London, 1991).

Pierrot, Jean, *The Decadent Imagination* (tr. Derek Coltman) (Chicago, 1981).

Pohlen, K., 'Kriminalstatistik betr. das RGBG', *Mitteilungen der Deutschen Gesellschaft zur Bekampfung der Geschlechtskrankheiten*, 31 (1933), 88–96.

Poller, Walter, *Arztschreiber in Buchenwald. Bericht des Häftlings 996 aus Block 39* (Hamburg, 1947).

Pompey, H., 'Gehirntod und totaler Tod. Moraltheologische Erwägungen zur Herztransplantation', *Münchener medizinische Wochenschrift*, 111 (1969), 736–41.

Porter, D. (ed.), *The History of Public Health and the Modern State* (Amsterdam, 1994).

Porter, R. & Porter, D., 'AIDS: Law, Liberty and Public Health' in Byrne, P. (ed.), *Health, Rights and Resources* (London, 1988), 76–93.

Porter, Roy, 'Quacks. An unconscionable time dying' in Budd, Susan & Sharma, Ursula (eds.), *The Healing Bond. The patient–practitioner relationship and therapeutic responsibility* (London & New York, 1994), 63–81.

Porter, Roy, *The Greatest Benefit to Mankind. A Medical History of Humanity from Antiquity to the Present* (London, 1997).

Power, H.J., 'Malaria, Drugs and World War II', paper presented 6 May 1994, *Malaria & War symposium*, Wellcome Institute for the History of Medicine, London.

Power, H.J., *Tropical Medicine in the Twentieth Century: A History of the Liverpool School of Tropical Medicine, 1898–1990* (London, 1999).

Praz, Mario, *The Romantic Agony* (New York, 1970).

Pribilla, O., 'Juristische, ärztliche und ethische Fragen zur Todesfeststellung', *Deutsches Ärzteblatt*, 65/41 (1968), 2256–59, 2318–22, 2396–98.

Probst, Christian, 'Die Religiosität des Landvolks im Urteil der Ärzte. Aus den Landes- und Volksbeschreibungen der bayerischen Amtsärzte um 1860', *Die Medizinische Welt*, 45 (1994), 152–56.

*Proceedings of the First International Conference on Sleeping sickness, London 17th of June 1907* (London, 1907), Cd 3778.

*Proceedings of the Imperial Social Hygiene Congress at the British Empire Exhibition, May 12th–16th, 1924* (London, 1924).

Pross, Christian, 'Die "Machtergreifung" am Krankenhaus' in Pross, Christian & Winau, Rolf (eds.), *Nicht mißhandeln!* (Stätten der Geschichte Berlins, Vol. 5) (Berlin, 1984), 180–205.

Pross, Christian, 'Die "Machtergreifung" im Krankenhaus' in Bleker, Johanna & Jachertz, Norbert (eds.), *Medizin im "Dritten Reich"* (Cologne, 1993), 97–108.

Pross, Christian & Winau, Rolf (eds.), *Nicht mißhandeln!* (Stätten der Geschichte Berlins, Vol. 5) (Berlin, 1984).

Prüll, Cay-Rüdiger (with assistance of Woodward, John) (ed.), *Pathology in the 19th and 20th Centuries. The Relationship between Theory and Practice* (Sheffield, 1997).

Prüll, Cay-Rüdiger, 'Aschoff, Ludwig' in Eckart, Wolfgang U. & Gradmann, Christoph (eds.), *Ärzte-Lexikon. Von der Antike bis zum 20. Jahrhundert* (München, 1995), 24–25.

Prüll, Cay-Rüdiger, 'Der Umgang mit der menschlichen Leiche: Medizinhistorischer Überblick' (unpublished paper presented at the conference 'Zum Umgang mit der Leiche in der Medizin' of the AEM (*Akademie für Ethik in der Medizin e.V.*) on July 8–9, 1994 in Heidelberg.

Prüll, Cay-Rüdiger, 'Die Sektion als letzter Dienst am Vaterland. Die deutsche "Kriegspathologie" im Ersten Weltkrieg' in Eckart, Wolfgang U. & Gradmann, Christoph (eds.), *Die Medizin und der Erste Weltkrieg* (Neuere Medizin- und Wissenschaftsgeschichte. Quellen und Studien, Vol. 3) (Pfaffenweiler, 1996), 155–82.

Prüll, Cay-Rüdiger, *Medizin am Lebenden oder am Toten? – Pathologie in Berlin und in London 1900 bis 1945* (Freiburg-im-Breisgau, forthcoming).

Quétel, C., *History of Syphilis* (Cambridge, 1990).

Raffalovich, André, 'Unisexualité anglaise', *Archives de l'anthropologie criminelle*, 11 (1896), 431.

Rahner, K., 'Theologische Erwägungen über den Eintritt des Todes' in Rahner, K., *Schriften zur Theologie*. Vol. IX, 2nd. ed. (Einsiedeln, Zürich, Köln, 1972), 323–35.

Rahner, K., *Schriften zur Theologie*. Vol. IX, 2nd. ed. (Einsiedeln, Zürich, Köln, 1972).

Ramsey, Matthew, 'The Politics of Professional Monopoly in Nineteenth-Century Medicine: The French Model and Its Rivals' in Geison, Gerald L. (ed.), *Professions and the French State* (Philadelphia, 1984), 225–305.

Ramsey, Matthew, *Professional and Popular Medicine in France, 1770–1830: The social world of medical practice* (Cambridge, 1988).

Reagan, Leslie J., *When Abortion was a Crime. Women, Medicine, and Law in the United States, 1867–1973* (Berkeley, Los Angeles & London, 1997).

Reese, Dagmar, Rosenhaft, Eve, Sachse, Carola & Siegel, Tilla (eds.), *Rationale Beziehungen? Geschlechterverhältnisse im Rationalisierungsprozeß* (Frankfurt/M., 1993).

Regin, C., *Selbsthilfe und Gesundsheitpolitik. Die Naturheilbewegung im Kaiserreich (1889 bis 1914)* (Stuttgart, 1995).

Reich, W.T. (ed.), *Encyclopedia of Bioethics* (revised edition, New York, 1995).

*Report of the 10th Parliamentary Committee on Population*, VDtRT, Vol. 411, No. 2714.

*Report of the 16th Parliamentary Committee on Population*, 7 July 1918, VDtRT, Vol. 321, No. 912.

*Report of the Committee of Inquiry on Venereal Disease* (London, 1923).

Retzlaff, I. & Wuermeling, H.-B. in Bockenheimer Lucius, G. & Seidler, E. (eds.), *Hirntod und Schwangerschaft. Dokumentation einer Diskussionsveranstaltung der Akademie für Ethik in der Medizin zum 'Erlanger Fall'* (Stuttgart, 1993).

Richardson, Ruth, *Death, Dissection and the Destitute* (London, 1988).

Rijksarchief Noord-Brabant ('s-Hertogenbosch), Archive *arrondissementsrechtbank Breda*.

Robertson, D.H.H. & George, G., 'Medical and Legal Problems in the Treatment of Delinquent Girls in Scotland', *British Journal of Venereal Diseases*, 46 (1970), 46–51.

Rogers, L., *Fevers in the Tropics* (Calcutta, 1907).

Rölleke, Heinz (ed.), *Georg Heym Lesebuch: Gedichte, Prosa, Träume, Tagebücher* (Munich, 1984).

Rollin, H.R, 'The Horton Malaria Laboratory, Epsom, Surrey (1925–1975)', *Journal of Medical Biography*, 2 (1994), 94–97.

Roseman, Mark (ed.), *Generations in Conflict. Youth revolt and generation formation in Germany 1770–1968* (Cambridge, 1995).

*Rotterdamsch Nieuwsblad.*

*Rotterdamsche Courant.*

Rotundo, E. Anthony, *American Manhood: Transformations from the Revolution to the Modern Era* (New York, 1993).

Ruff, W., *Organverpflanzung. Ethische Probleme aus katholischer Sicht* (München, 1971).

Ruggiero, Guido, 'The Cooperation of Physicians and the State in the Control of Violence in Renaissance Venice', *Journal of the History of Medicine and Allied Sciences*, 33, 156–66.

Ruggiero, Guido, *Violence in Early Renaissance Venice* (New Brunswick, NJ, 1980).


Sakr, L., et al., 'Zur hohen Autopsierate in Wien', *Wiener klinische Wochenschrift*, 101 (1989), 511–14.

Sanders, Ewoud & Tempelaars, Rob, *Krijg de vinkentering! 1001 Nederlandse en Vlaamse verwensingen* (Amsterdam & Antwerpen, 1998).

Sauerteig, L., 'Frauenemanzipation und Sittlichkeit. Die Rezeption des englischen Abolitionismus in Deutschland' in Muhs, R., Paulmann, J. & Steinmetz, W. (eds.), *Aneignung und Abwehr. Interkultureller Transfer zwischen Deutschland und Großbritannien im 19. Jahrhundert* (Bodenheim, forthcoming).

Sauerteig, L., 'Moralismus versus Pragmatismus: Die Kontroverse um Schutzmittel gegen Geschlechtskrankheiten zu Beginn des 20. Jahrhunderts im deutsch-englischen Vergleich', in Dinges, M. and Schlich, T. (eds), *Neue Wege in der Seuchengeschichte* (Stuttgart, 1995), 207–47.

Sauerteig, L., 'Vergleich: Ein Königsweg auch für die Medizingeschichte? Methodologische Fragen vergleichenden Forschens', in Paul, N. & Schlich, T. (eds.), *Medizingeschichte: Aufgaben, Probleme, Perspektiven* (Frankfurt/M. & New York, 1998).

Sauerteig, L., 'Sex, Medicine and Morality during the First World War' in Harrison, M. & Cooter, R. (eds), *War, Medicine and Modernity, 1860–1945* (Stroud, 1999).

Sauerteig, L., *Krankeit, Sexualität, Gesellschaft: Geschlechtskrankheiten und Gesundheitspolitik in Deutschland im 19. frühen 20. Jahrhundert* (Stuttgart, forthcoming)

Savitt, T.L., 'The Use of Blacks for Medical Experimentation and Demonstration in the Old South', *Journal of Southern History*, XLVIII (1982), 331–48.

Schäfer, Herbert, *Der Okkulttäter* (Hamburg, 1959).

Schattenfroh, Silvia, 'Wiederverwertung nach dem Tode. Organentnahme und Transplantation', *Frankfurter Allgemeine Zeitung*, March 1st, 1994, 14.

Schellong, S., *Künstliche Beatmung. Strukturgeschichte eines ethischen Dilemmas* (Stuttgart, 1990).

Schepper-Lambers, Friederike, *Beerdigungen und Friedhöfe im 19. Jahrhundert in Münster* (Beiträge zur Volkskultur in Nordwestdeutschland, Vol. 73).

Schettler, G., Gillmann, H., Ritz, E. et al., 'Indikationen und Kontraindikationen der Organtransplantation', *Studium Generale*, 23 (1970), 301–12.

Scheven, Katharina in *Der Abolitionist*, 7 (1908), 11–16

Schlich, T., 'Medizingeschichte und Ethik der Transplantationsmedizin: Die Erfindung der Organtransplantation', in: Albert, F.W., Land, W., & Zwierlein, W. E. (eds.), *Transplantationsmedizin und Ethik. Auf dem Weg zu einem gesellschaftlichen Konsens* (Lengerich & Berlin, 1994), 11–32.

Schlich, T., 'Die Geschichte der Herztransplantation. Chirurgie, Wissenschaft, Ethik', in Frewer, A., Köhler, M. & Rödel, C.(eds.), *Herztransplantation und Ethik. Historische und philosophische Aspekte eines paradigmatischen Eingriffs der modernen Medizin* (Erlangen, Jena (Erlanger Studien zur Ethik in der Medizin, Bd. 4), 1996), 13–38.

Schlich, T., *Die Erfindung der Organtransplantation. Erfolg und Scheitern des chirurgischen Organersatzes (1880–1930)* (Frankfurt & New York, 1998).

Schmölder, R., 'Strafrechtliche und civilrechtliche Bedeutung der Geschlechtskrankheiten', *Zeitschrift für Bekämpfung der Geschlechtskrankheiten*, 1 (1903), 73–94.

Schneider, H., 'Der Hirntod. Begriffsgeschichte und Pathogenese', *Der Nervenarzt*, 41 (1970), 381–87.

Schnitzer, R.J. & Hawking, F., *Experimental chemotherapy* (New York, 1963).

Schulte, Regina, 'Infanticide in rural Bavaria in the nineteenth century' in Medick, Hans & Sabean, David Warren (eds.), *Interest and emotion. Essays on the study of family and kinship* (Cambridge, 1984), 77–102.

Schupbach, W., 'Sequah; an English "American medicine"-man in 1890', *Medical History*, 29 (1985), 272–317.

Schütze, C., 'Herzchirurgie mit offenen Fragen', *Süddeutsche Zeitung*, No. 12, 13./14. Jan. 1968, 13.

Scottish Record Office, HH65/122/60, *Evidence of Scottish Covenant Association to Royal Commission on Scottish Affairs*, 22 Oct. 1953.

Seesemann, Heinrich, 'Ist eine heimliche Leichensektion strafbar?', *Ärztliches Vereinsblatt*, 55 (1928), 721.

Seesemann, Heinrich, 'Ist eine heimliche Leichensektion strafbar?', *Ärztliches Vereinsblatt*, 60 (1931).

Seidler, Eduard, 'Pathologie in Freiburg', *Beiträge zur Allgemeinen Pathologie und pathologischen Anatomie*, 158 (1976), 9–22.

Seidler, Eduard, *Die Medizinische Fakultät der Albert-Ludwigs-Universität Freiburg im Breisgau. Grundlagen und Entwicklungen* (Berlin & Heidelberg, 1991).

Seiffert, K.E., 'Überblick über den gegenwärtigen Stand der Transplantation von Organen und Geweben', *Der Chirurg*, 38 (1967), 255–59.

*Sequah archives*, CMAC, Wellcome Insitute for the History of Medcine.

Selberg, Torunn, 'Personal narratives on healing', *Fabula* 31 (1990) 284–88.

Shields, D., 'War Conditions and Venereal Disease: The Recent Ministry Circular', ibid., 159–60; Fawcett Library, AMSH 310/1, Ministry of Health, 'Circular No 2727', 8 January 1943.

Sicroff, Albert, *Les controverses des status de "pureté de sang" en Espagne du XVe au XVIIe siècles* (Paris, 1960).

Sighele, Scipio, *Litterature et criminalité* (Paris, 1908).

Silverman, Deborah L., *Art Nouveau in Fin-de-Siècle France* (Berkeley, 1989).

Sittner, G., 'Wir werden keine Jagd auf Spender machen', *Süddeutsche Zeitung*, No. 40, 15/16 Feb. 1969, 3.

Sittner, G., 'Am Blutpfropf scheiterte die Verpflanzung', *Süddeutsche Zeitung*, No. 41, 17 Feb. 1969, 3.

Smith, F. B., 'The Contagious Diseases Acts Reconsidered', *Social History of Medicine*, 3 (1990), 197–215.

Soden, Kristine von, 'Paragraph 218 – streichen, nicht ändern! 'Abtreibung und Geburtenregelung in der Weimarer Republik' in Deutsches Hygiene Museum, Dresden (ed.), *Unter anderen Umständen. Zur Geschichte der Abtreibung* (Berlin, 1993).

Solomon, Susan Gross, 'The Health of the Other: Medical Research and Empire in 1920s Russia' in Woodward, John & Jütte, Robert (eds.), *Coping with Sickness. Perspectives on Health Care, Past and Present Perspectives on Health Care, Past and Present* (Sheffield, 1996), 137–60.

Solloway, Frank J., *Freud: Biologist of the Mind* (New York, 1979).

Spann, W. & Liebhardt, E.W., 'Reanimation und Feststellung des Todeszeitpunktes', *Münchener medizinische Wochenschrift*, 108 (1966), 1410–14.

Spann, W., 'Allgemeine Diskussion' in Krösl, W. & Scherzer E. (eds.), *Die Bestimmung des Todeszeitpunktes. Kongreß in der Wiener Hofburg vom 4. bis 6. Mai 1972* (Wien, 1973), 339–62.

Spann, W., 'Strafrechtliche Probleme an der Grenze von Leben und Tod', *Deutsche Zeitschrift für die gesamte gerichtliche Medizin*, 57 (1966), 26–30.

Spann, W., Kugler, J., & Liebhardt, E.W., 'Tod und elektrische Stille im EEG', *Münchener medizinische Wochenschrift*, 42 (1967), 2161–67.

Spicker, S.F et al. (eds.), *The Use of Human Beings in Research with Special Reference to Clinical Trials* (Dordrecht, Boston & London, 1988).

Spongberg, M., *Feminizing Venereal Disease: The Body of the Prostitute in Nineteenth-Century Medical Discourse* (London, 1997).

St. Vincent de Paroism, M.J.F.A. de, *Du dépecage criminel* (Lyon, 1902).

Staden, Heinrich von, 'The Discovery of the Body: Human Dissection and its cultural Contexts in Ancient Greece', *The Yale Journal of Biology and Medicine*, 65 (1992), 223–41.

Stapenhorst, K.,'Über die biologisch-naturwissenschaftlich unzulässige Gleichsetzung von Hirntod und Individualtod und ihre Folgen für die Medizin', *Ethik in der Medizin*, 8 (1996), 79–98.

Stark, T., *Knife to the Heart: the Story of Transplant Surgery* (London, 1996).

Starr, P., *The Social Transformation of American Medicine* (New Haven, 1982).

Stephens, J.W.W., 'Studies in the Treatment of Malaria XXXII: Summary of Studies I – XXXI', *Annals of Tropical Medicine and Parasitology*, 17 (1923), 303–05.

Stephens, J.W.W., Yorke, W., Blacklock, B., Macfie, J.W.S., & Cooper, C.F., 'Studies in the Treatment of Malaria', *Annals of Tropical Medicine and Parasitology*, 11 (1917–18), 91–111.

Stiffoni, Giovanni et al., *La época de los primeros borbones II. La cultura española entre el Barroco y la Ilustración (1680–1759)* (Madrid, 1988).

Stockel, S., *Sauglingsfursorge zwisischen sozialer Hygiene und Eugenik. Das Beispiel Berlins im Kaiserreich und in der Weimarer Republik* (Berlin & New York, 1996).

Surgeon General's Office, *The Index-Catalogue of the Library of the Surgeon General's Office.*

Svendsen, Einar, 'Autopsy Legislation and Practice in Various Countries', *Archive of Pathology and Laboratory Medicine*, 111 (1987), 846–50.

Swazey, J.P. & Fox, R.C., 'The Clinical Moratorium' in Fox, R.C. (ed.), *Essays in Medical Sociology. Journeys into the Field* (New York, 1979), 325–63.


Tarde, Gabriel, *The Laws of Imitation* (New York, 1903).

Tarde, Gabriel, *Penal Philosophy* (Boston, 1912).

*The Chemist and Druggist.*

*The Greenock Herald.*

*The Medical Officer.*

The Public Health (Venereal Diseases) Regulation, 1916, 12 July 1916, *Statutory Rules and Orders* (1916), Vol. 3, 74–76.

Thielecke, H., 'Das Recht des Menschen auf seinen Tod', *Fortschritte der Medizin*, 86 (1968), 1067–68.

Thielecke, H., *Wer darf leben? Ethische Probleme der modernen Medizin* (München, 1970).

Thoinot, L. & Weysse, A.W., *Medicolegal Aspects of Moral Offenses* (Philadelphia, 1921).

Thomas, H.W., 'The Experimental Treatment of Trypanosomiasis in Animals', *Proceedings of the Royal Society, Series B*, LXXVI (1905), 589–91.

Tibbits, D. R., *The Medical, Social and Political Response to Venereal Diseases in Victoria 1860–1980* (Ph.D. dissertation, Monash University, 1994).

Tomás y Valiente, Francisco, 'Relaciones de la Inquisición con el aparato institucional del Estado', in Pérez Villanueva, Joaquín (ed.), *La Inquisición española. Nueva visión, nuevos horizontes* (Madrid, 1980), 41–60.

Toulouse, Édouard, *Le Rapport des médicins expert sur Vacher* (Clermont, 1898).

Toulouse, Édouard, *Les Conflits intersexuelles et sociaux* (Paris, 1904).

Towers, B.A., 'Health Education Policy 1916–1926: Venereal Disease and the Prophylaxis Dilemma', *Medical History*, 24 (1980), 70–87.

Trockel, H., 'Rechtliche Probleme der Organtransplantation', *Medizinische Klinik*, 64 (1969), 666–68.


Überfuhr, P., Reichart, B., Welz, A. et al., 'Bericht über eine erfolgreiche orthotope Herztransplantation in Deutschland', *Klinische Wochenschrift*, 60 (1982), 1435–42.

Unschuld, Paul, 'The Conceptual Determination (Überformung) of Individual and Collective Experiences of Illness' in Currer, Caroline & Stacey, Margaret (eds.), *Concepts of Health, Illness and Disease. Comparative Perspective* (Providence & Oxford, 1986).

Usborne, Cornelie, *The Politics of the Body in Weimar Germany. Women's reproductive rights and duties* (London & Ann Arbor, 1992).

Usborne, Cornelie, *The Cultures of Abortion in Weimar & Nazi Germany* (forthcoming).

Usborne, Cornelie, 'The New Woman and generation conflict: perceptions of young women's sexual mores in the Weimar Republic' in Roseman, Mark (ed.), *Generations in Conflict. Youth revolt and generation formation in Germany 1770–1968* (Cambridge, 1995), 137–63.

Usborne, Cornelie, 'Wise women, wise men and abortion in the Weimar Republic: gender, class and medicine' in Abrams, L. & Harvey, E. (eds.), *Gender Relations in German History* (London, 1996), 143–76.

Usborne, Cornelie, 'Abortion for sale! The competition between quacks and doctors in Weimar Germany' in Gijswijt-Hofstra, Marijke, Marland, Hilary & Witt, Hans de (eds.), *Illness and Healing Alternatives in Western Europe* (London, 1997), 183–204.

Usborne, Cornelie & de Blecourt, Willem, 'Pains of the past. Recent Research in the Social History of Medicine in Germany', *Bulletin of the German Historical Institute*, 21 (1999), 5–21.

Uthman, Edward O., *The Routine Autopsy. The Procedure related in narrative Form. A Guide for Screenwriters and Novelists* (uthman@neosoft.com).

Uzanne, Octave, *Idées sur les romans, par D.A.F. Sade* (Paris, 1878).


Valiente, Francisco Tomás y, *La tortura en España. Estudios históricos* (Barcelona, 1973).

Valiente, Francisco Tomás y, 'El proceso penal', *Historia 16. Extra I* (Diciembre 1976), 19–35.

van Riel, J., 'Geschiedkundig overzicht der Vereeniging over de jaren 1880–1905' in *Gedenkboek van de Vereeniging tegen de kwakzalverij* (Dordrecht, 1906), 160–97.

Vasold, Manfred, *Rudolf Virchow. Der große Arzt und Politiker* (Stuttgart, 1988).

Vaughan, M., *Curing Their Ills: Colonial Power and African Illness* (Cambridge, 1991).

Vekene, E. Van der, *Bibliotheca Bibliographica Historia Sanctae Inquisitionis*, 2 Vols. (Vacluz, 1982).

*Verfahren bei der Behandlung der in dem Charité-Krankenhause Verstorbenen, insbesondere Sektionen; Dezember 1929 bis März 1938*, Bundesarchiv Berlin. Abteilung Lichterfelde (BArchiv Berlin), Reichsministerium für Wissenschaft, Erziehung und Volksbildung.

*Verfahren bei der Behandlung der in dem Charité-Krankenhause Verstorbenen, insbesondere Sektionen, Dezember 1929 bis März 1938* in Bundesarchiv Berlin, Reichsministerium für Wissenschaft, Erziehung und Volksbildung, Bd.2, Nr.2697.

Vincke, Johannes (ed.), *Freiburger Professoren des 19. und 20. Jahrhunderts* (Freiburg i. Br., 1957).

Virchow, Rudolf, 'Das Pathologische Institut' in Guttstadt, Albert (ed.), *Die naturwissenschaftlichen und medicinischen Staatsanstalten Berlins. Festschrift für die 59. Versammlung deutscher Naturforscher und Aerzte* (Berlin, 1886), pp. 288–300.

Vogel, H.-J., 'Zustimmung oder Widerspruch. Bemerkungen zu einer Kernfrage der Organtransplantation', *Neue juristische Wochenschrift*, 33/12 (1980), 625–29.

*Volkskunde-atlas voor Nederland en Vlaams-België*, *Commentaar*, II (Antwerpen, 1965).

Vollman, J. & Winau, R, 'Informed Consent in Human Experimentation Before the Nuremberg Code', *British Medical Journal*, 313 (1996), 1445–47.

Vollmann, J., 'Medizinische Probleme des Hirntodkriteriums', *Medizinische Klinik*, 91 (1996), 39–45.


Waddington, I., *The Medical Profession in the Industrial Revolution* (Dublin, 1984).

Walkowitz, J.R., *Prostitution and Victorian Society. Women, Class, and the State* (Cambridge, 1980).

Walter, Roland, *Die Leichenschau und das Sektionswesen. Grundzpüge der Entwicklung von ihren Anfängen bis zu den Bemühungen um eine einheitliche Gesetzgebung* (Thesis, Med. Fac., Düsseldorf, 1971).

Walther, D.,'Theologisch-ethische Aspekte einer Herztransplantation' in Honecker, M. (ed.), *Aspekte und Probleme der Organverpflanzung* (Neukirchen-Vluyn, 1973), 19–32.

Wawersik, J., 'Kriterien des Todes', *Studium Generale*, 23 (1970), 319–30.

Wear, A., French, R.K. & Lonie, I.M. (eds.), *The medical renaissance of the sixteenth-century* (Cambridge, 1985).

Wear, A., Geyer-Kordesch, J. & French, R. (eds.), *Doctors and Ethics: The Earlier Historical Setting of Professional Ethics* (Amsterdam & Atlanta, 1993).

Weatherall, D., *Medicine and the Quiet Art: Medical Research and Patient Care* (Oxford, 1995).

Weindling, P., *Health, Race and German Politics Between National Unification and Nazism, 1870–1945* (Cambridge, 1989).

Weindling, P., 'Sexually Transmitted Diseases between Imperial and Nazi Germany', *Genitourinary Medicine*, 70 (1994), 284–85.

Weiss, B., *Rezeption der Einwände von Hans Jonas gegen die Feststellung des Hirntodes als Tod des Menschen* (Diss. med., Erlangen, 1991).

White, B., 'Training *ve* Medical Policemen: Forensic Medicine and Public Health in Nineteenth-Century Scotland', in Clark, M. & Crawford, C. (eds.), *Legal Medicine in History* (Cambridge, 1994), 145–63.

White, L., '"They Could Make Their Victims Dull": Genders and Genres, Fantasies and Cures in Colonial Southern Uganda', *American Historical Review* (1995), 1379–1402.

Wiesemann, C., 'Instrumentalisierte Instrumente: EEG, zerebrale Angiographie und die Etablierung des Hirntod-Konzepts' in Meinel, C. (ed.), *Instrument – Experiment* (Berlin, 2000).

Wiesemann, C., 'Hirntod und Gesellschaft. Argumente für einen pragmatischen Skeptizismus', *Ethik in der Medizin*, 6 (1995), 16–28.

Wiesemann, C., 'Medizin und reflexive Modernisierung am Beispiel der Hirntod-Kontroverse' in Hohlfeld, R. & Lau, C. (eds.), *Wissenschaft und reflexive Modernisierung* (Finck, 1998).

Willcox, R.R., 'Fifty Years Since the Conception of an Organized Venereal Diseases Service in Great Britain. The Royal Commission of 1916', *British Journal of Venereal Disease*, 43 (1967), 1–9.

Wissenschaftlicher Beirat der Bundesärztekammer, 'Kriterien des Hirntodes. Entscheidungshilfen zur Feststellung des Hirntodes', *Deutsches Ärzteblatt*, 79 (1982), (C) 35–41.

Wolf, Friedrich, *Cyankali. Woman as Sexual Criminal* (New York, 1934).

Woodward, John & Jütte, Robert (eds.), *Coping with Sickness: Perspectives on Health Care, Past and Present* (Sheffield, 1996).

Woodward, John, 'Health Care, Past and Present' in Woodward, John & Jütte, Robert (eds.), *Coping with Sickness: Perspectives on Health Care, Past and Present* (Sheffield, 1996), 1–13.

Woycke, James, *Birth Control in Germany 1871–1933* (London, 1988).

Wuermeling, H.-B., 'Gefährliches Nachdenken über anencephale Neugeborene als Organspender', *Medizinische Ethik. Sonderbeilage des Ärzteblatt Baden-Württemberg*, 4/27 (1988).

Yerushalmi, Y., *From Spanish Court to Italian Ghetto: Isaac Cardoso. A Study in Seventeenth-Century Marranism and Jewish Apologetics* (New York, 1971).

Zaner, R.M. (ed.), *Death: Beyond Whole-brain Criteria* (Dordrecht, 1988).

Zenker, R. & Pichlmaier, H., 'Organverpflanzung beim Menschen', *Deutsche medizinische Wochenschrift*, 93 (1968), 713–20.

Zenker, R., Klinner, W., Sebening, F. et al., 'Herztransplantation – Möglichkeiten und Problematik', *Münchener medizinische Wochenschrift*, 111 (1969), 749–54.

# Index

Aberdeen, 137, 139
abortions, 4, 91–103
Accra, 112, 114, 121
Acts of Parliament, 40, 76, 128–30, 132, 133, 135–37, 139, 140, 157, 159
advertising, 78
Africa, 5, 107–21, 151, 152
alcohol & alcoholism, 59, 66, 69
Algemeen Handelsblad, 85
alternative medicine, 81, 95
America, 2, 65, 110, 152, 157
Amsterdam, 78, 86
anarchism, 57, 61
anatomy, 31, 99
    departments of, 36
    morbid, 3, 31, 32, 40, 41
    pathological, 31–35, 41
Andalusia, 18
anthropology, 6, 41, 64, 154
    criminal, 59, 60
anthropometry, 60
apothecaries, 11, 14, 20
Aragon, 18
arsenic, 110
artificial respiration, 149, 151, 155
*Ärztliches Vereinsblatt*, 43
Aschoff, Ludwig, 30, 40–42
asylums, 57, 58, 60, 113
atheism, 62
atoxyl, 110

attitudes
    changing, 81
    conservative, 97
    legal, 91
    of physicians & practitioners, 34
    of practitioners in court, 22
    of women, 93
    social, 137, 150, 151
    to death, 35
    to health care, 120
    to sexuality, 137
Auschwitz, 38
Australia, 139
Austria, 30
autonomy, 39, 107, 121, 139
autopsies, 3, 29–43
*autos-da-fé*, 20

Baden, 36
barbers, 13, 15, 20
Barcelona, 15
Barnard, Christiaan, 151–53, 156, 157
Baudelaire, 61
Bay, Eberhard, 153
Bayer 205, 117–19
Bayly, Hugh Wansy, 132
Beck, Ulrich, 150, 158, 159
beliefs
    about death, 32, 159
    mystical, 33
    of lower-class women, 95

popular, 33, 159
religious, 32, 33
traditional, 32, 33, 39, 41, 42
Beller, Fritz K., 158
Berlin, 32, 35, 38, 94, 95, 97, 100, 101,
   103, 129
   Charité-Hospital, 31, 34, 35
   Rudolf Virchow Hospital, 38
   Rudolf Virchow Institute, 40
Berlin University, 31, 32, 35, 39
*Berliner Zeitung*, 34
bigamy, 3, 22
Bijsterveldt, 82
Binet, Alfred, 62, 63, 65
bio-ethics, 6, 7
birth control, 92, 95
birth rate, 68, 92
Blackett, Sir Basil, 133
Blacklock, Donald, 115
Blaiberg, Philip, 152, 156
Blaschko, Alfred, 129
blasphemy, 3, 16, 22
Bockelmann, Paul, 155
Böckle, Franz, 153, 157
Bond, Charles J., 133, 134
Borja, Cardinal, 21
BR 68, 117
brain death, 5, 149–60
Breinl, Anton, 110
British Social Hygiene Council, 133
Brown, Ernest, 135
Buchenwald, 38

Cardano, 13
Castile, 13, 18
Catholicism, 3, 18, 22, 34, 69, 93, 129,
   153
Cave, Sir George, 132
Centre Party (Zentrum), 129
Charité-Hospital, 39
charms, 19, 69, 103
chemotherapy, 109, 110, 112, 117

childbirth, 92
China, 38
cholera, 128
Christ, 56, 84–86
Christian churches, 33
Christian ideology, 86
Christianity, 18
Church of England, 138
Church of Scotland, 138
circumcision, 17
civil code, 36
civil liberties, 140
civil rights, 96
clientele, 14
clinical examinations, 29, 32, 112
clinical medicine, 108, 121
clinical practice, 32, 108, 117, 120, 149
clinical trials, 108, 114, 117, 120
code of conduct, 16
code of ethics, 16
code of practice, 17
coercion, 132, 140
Colonial Medical Department, 115
Colonial Medical Service, 114, 115
colonial medicine, 109, 116, 119, 120
colonialism, 120
coma, 155
communication
   between healer and patient, 82–84
   of infections, 129, 135, 137
compulsory notification, 128–35, 139
concentration camps, 38
confidentiality, 128, 130, 140
consent, 3, 108, 114, 120, 156–59
   informed, 42, 107, 108
   of relatives, 29, 30, 35, 38
contraception, 92
Conversos, 12, 18–21
corpses, 31, 32, 33, 34, 35, 36, 37, 41
   acquisition of, 37
   examination of, 29, 36
   handling of, 35, 37

Corson, J.F., 117–19
court physicians, 15
Court, German Imperial, 36, 37, 39
courts, 4, 12–15, 17, 19, 21, 22, 36–38, 56, 58, 59, 78, 86, 91–103, 138. *See also* trials
crime, 4, 59, 68, 69, 91, 92, 102
    fight against, 3, 13, 22
    of passion, 57
criminal anthropology, 59, 60
criminal law, 4, 91, 94, 132, 155
criminal psychiatry, 59
criminality, 59, 69
criminals, 31, 59, 60, 61, 68, 69
Cruz, Francisco de la, 21
Crypto-Judaism, 3, 17
culture, 29, 59, 93, 96, 111, 139
cyclosporin, 156

Darwall, Denise, 151, 153
Davenport, Charles A., 77–86
Dawson, Lord, 133
de Sade, 55, 61, 63
death, 5, 30, 37, 62, 99, 101, 152, 153. *See also* brain death *and* maternal mortality
    attitudes to, 35
    beliefs about, 32, 159
    cause of, 29, 32, 38, 40, 96
    certification of, 15
    concept of, 152
    definition of, 149, 151–55, 157, 159
    life after, 32, 42
    of patients, 29, 31, 38, 153
death penalty, 20, 59
decadence, 55, 61, 62
Defence of the Realm Regulations, 132, 135, 136
deification, 84
denouncement, 19–21, 95
depopulation, 68
*Der Spiegel*, 151, 153, 157, 159
detection rate, 91

*Die Welt*, 151, 152
discipline, 135, 138
Dordrecht, 84, 85
dosages, 5, 109, 112–14, 116, 117, 119, 120
Dostoievski, 62
drug regimes, 112, 113
drug tests, 5, 107–21
druggists, 20

eating habits, 17
Eckart, Wolfgang, 110
education, 35, 77, 81, 93, 115, 128, 131, 133–35
EEG, 155
Ehrlich, Paul, 109
emancipation, 92
embalmments, 13
emetine, 115, 116
England, 62, 64, 78, 128, 130–35, 137, 140
*ens morbi*, 32
Erlangen, 159
ethnic minorities, 110
Eugenics, 39, 138
euthanasia, 38
exhibitionism, 55, 63
experiments, 5, 38, 107–09, 114, 118, 120, 121
expulsion, 18

family planning, 100
*féminisme*, 67
fertility, 69, 92
*fin de siècle*, 4, 56, 62, 69, 86
Flaubert, 61
foetus, 100, 103
Forssmann, Werner, 153, 154
fortune telling, 94–96, 103
France, 30, 55, 62, 63, 66, 67, 69, 95, 138, 155
Franz II, Emperor, 30

Freetown, 110, 115
Freiburg, 30, 40, 43
funerals, 33, 36, 37, 150, 156

Galen, 15, 17
Galenism, 19, 21
gender, 2, 4–6, 63, 65–68, 70, 81, 91, 101, 102, 120, 128
German Democratic Republic, 30
German Empire, 36, 40
German Medical Academy, Shanghai, 38
German Parliament. *See* Reichstag
German Society for Combating VD, 129, 130
German Society for Neurosurgery, 153
German Society of Surgery, 153, 155
germanin, 117, 119
Germany, 2, 3, 5, 29–43, 62, 68, 91–103, 128–30, 138–40, 149–60
Germany, Federal Republic of, 39
Ghana, 112
Giessen, 41
Gold Coast, 112
Gordon, Rupert, 115, 116
gout, 17
Government, 33, 36, 38, 40, 115, 116, 121, 131, 132, 135, 137, 157
Granada, 15, 20
Great Britain, 2, 5, 30, 31, 110, 111, 114, 131, 134, 135
Groningen, 86
guilt, 15, 16, 69
gynaecology, 101, 158

haematobium, 115, 116
Hague, The, 80, 86
Hamburg, 128, 152, 154
Harrison, Colonel L.W., 134
healers, 2, 4, 11, 12, 18, 19, 75–84, 86, 95, 128
*Health & Empire*, 133

health care, 3, 14, 42, 107, 120
health education, 128, 131, 133, 135
health insurance, 95
heart, 18, 116, 149, 151–53, 155–58
Hebrew, 14
Heinemann, Gustav, 154
Henoch, Eduard, 32
Herzog, Georg, 41
heterosexuality, 66
Hippocrates, 15
historiography, 31
Histotom, 38
Holland. *See* Netherlands
Holocaust, 6
Holy Office, 3, 11, 12–1719, 22
homosexuality, 61, 63, 66–68
honour, 12, 14, 15
hospitalisation, 15, 57, 112–15
human experimentation, 107–09, 120
human rights, 2, 3, 6, 7, 30, 34, 40, 42, 107, 108
hygiene
    moral, 136
    racial, 39
    social, 127, 133, 136, 138, 139
hysteria, 68

Ikoma, 117
illegitimacy, 101
immorality, 59, 93
income, 14
infamy, 19
infanticide, 4, 91, 100
Ingrassia, 13
injections, 113, 115–17
injury, 96, 99, 101, 109, 118, 159
Inquisition, Spanish, 2, 11–22
intensive care, 151, 158
intimidation, 57, 63, 92, 94, 95, 97
inversion, 55, 57, 65, 67

Jadassohn, Joseph, 130

Jews, 3, 17–22
Jiama, 115
Johnstone, Ralph W., 131
judges, 12, 15, 58, 68, 94, 97, 101, 102
judiciary, 93, 97

Kantrowitz, Adrian, 151, 158
Kautzky, Rudolph, 152
kidneys, 77, 119, 151, 153, 156
Kleine, Professor F.K., 117
Königsberg, 37
Konno, 115
Korro, 115, 116, 121
Krafft-Ebing, Richard von, 63, 64, 66

Lacassagne, Alexandre, 59–62, 64,
    66–69
language, 17, 82, 83, 93, 97, 155, 157
law
    abortion, 92, 97, 99, 102
    and medicine, 3, 4, 6, 12, 13, 29,
        86, 127, 138, 140, 151. *See also*
        legal medicine
    and morality, 5, 128, 140
    and quackery, 4, 75, 76, 86
    and sexuality, 5, 128, 140
    autopsy, 3, 29–43
    breaking of, 12, 13
    common, 137
    courts of. *See* courts
    criminal, 4, 91, 94, 132, 155
    enforcement, 93, 97, 103
    immigration, 78
    licensing, 75
    penal, 38, 129
    reform, 4, 91, 92, 102, 129
    sexually-transmitted diseases,
        127–40
    transplantation, 159
lawyers, 5, 14, 80, 97, 140, 149,
    154–57, 159, 160
League of Human Rights, 34
League of Nations, 117
Lees, Dr David, 138

legal
    arguments, 76
    attitudes, 91
    coercion, 140
    compulsion, 5, 127, 135
    controls, 132
    definition, 120
    documents, 95
    experts, 37
    ideology, 137
    language, 98
    medicine, 13, 59–61, 65, 69
    policies, 149
    privileges, 15, 22
    procedures, 15
    process, 138
    regulations, 2, 3, 12, 29, 30, 35, 37,
        39, 42
    security, 14
    situation, 3, 35, 37, 39, 42
    solutions, 151
    system, 36, 86, 137
        loopholes in, 78
    traditions, 13
legislation
    autopsy, 3, 29, 30, 39, 42
    emergency, 129
    infectious diseases, 128
    public health, 5, 128
    venereal disease, 129, 136
Leibnitz, Wilhelm von, 1
*Leichenordnungen*, 36
*Leichenschau*, 36
Lenz, Fritz, 39
Liszt, Franz von, 129
Liverpool, 107–21, 140
    Royal Infirmary, 111
    School of Tropical Medicine,
        110–12, 114, 115, 117
Local Government Board, 130, 131
Lombroso, Cesare, 59
loopholes, 86
López, Gaspar, 17
Lubarsch, Otto, 35, 36
Lucifer, 94

Madrid, 20, 21
magic, 19, 33, 103
   sympathetic, 95, 96, 103
magnetic sympathy, 95
malaria, 110–15
Maria Theresia, 30
Martindale, Dr W., 115
masculinity, 55, 63–69
masochism, 55, 63–65, 68
masturbation, 56, 63
maternal mortality, 99
May, Otto, 132
medical
   advice, 135, 136
   associations, 4, 86, 93, 157
   care, 1–3, 15, 19, 42, 95, 114
   circles, 21
   controls, 130
   costs, 14
   council, 101
   debate, 128
   doctrines, 19
   education, 32, 35, 75
   establishment, 22
   evaluation, 16
   evidence, 15–17
   examinations, 16, 17, 131, 132, 135, 136
   expertise, 13, 15, 22, 58–60, 97, 101, 138, 150
   faculty, 15, 35, 39, 80
   ideology, 137
   inspections, 78, 130, 137
   law. *See* law and medicine
   licensing, 75
   monopoly, 80
   organisations, 156
   policies, 149
   practice, 2, 7, 11, 19, 32, 120
   practitioners, 2, 11–22, 75, 130. *See also* practitioners
   prestige, 82
   profession, 1–4, 12, 33, 78, 91, 99, 129, 134, 153, 156, 157
   progress, 5, 35, 158, 160
   reports, 16
   research, 108, 110
   schools, 75
   science, 17, 140, 150, 156, 158, 160
   scientists, 67, 149, 152, 154
   students, 20, 41
   success, 99
   system, 19
   texts, 13
   training, 76
   treatment, 135
   works, 15, 21
Medical Department, 110, 115
Medical Officers, 117, 131, 132, 137, 138, 140
Medical Research Council, 111, 117
medicalisation, 55, 92, 94
Médici, Catherine de, 65
medicine, 1, 2, 7, 17, 19, 22, 31, 58, 75, 76, 80, 99, 108, 110, 119, 121, 140, 152, 154, 156
   academic, 19
   alternative, 81, 95
   and law, 3, 4, 6, 12, 13, 29, 86, 127, 138, 140, 151. *See also* legal medicine
   and morality, 127–40
   clinical, 108, 121
   colonial, 109, 116, 119, 120
   experimental, 120, 121
   folk, 137
   forensic, 36
   history of, 4, 7, 41, 91
   illegal practice of, 86
   in universities, 15, 22, 32
   intensive care, 151, 158
   legal. *See* legal medicine
   orthodox, 19
   Romantic, 31
   scientific, 31–35, 40–42
   tropical, 110, 111, 117, 120. *See also* Liverpool School of Tropical Medicine
medicines, 14, 78, 79, 115, 116
Medinaceli, Duke of, 21
mental deficiency, 61, 136
mental health, 16, 57, 59

mental illness, 34
mental irresponsibility, 58
Mercurialis, 13
midwifery, 99
Ministry of Health, 131, 133–36, 139
Ministry of Justice, 157
Ministry of Law, 35
Ministry of Science, 34, 35, 39
minority, 12, 18, 110, 132, 140
miscarriage, 100
misconduct, 101
misfortune, 76, 94, 103
misogyny, 65
modernisation, 5, 6, 150, 152, 153,
    158–60
modernity, 95, 150, 151, 156, 158, 160
monarchy, 12, 18
Mond, Sir Alfred, 134
monopoly, 4, 91
moral
    decay, 127
    education, 132
    egoism, 69
    hygiene, 136
    imbeciles, 61, 136
    limits, 149
    order, 137
    panic, 136
    policy, 138
    problems, 154
    standards, 153
    theology, 153
morality, 127–40
Moriscos, 3, 18, 19, 22
Munich, 153, 155, 157
Muñoz y Peralta, Juan, 21
murder, 56, 60, 66, 69, 92
music, 76, 77, 79–81, 83, 84
Muslims, 14, 18

Nájera, Felipe de, 17
nakedness, 55, 79, 83
Napoleon, 75, 128

National Council for Combating VD,
    131–33
National Council of Women, 139
national identity, 139
National Socialism, 38
nationalism, 139
*Naturgeschichte*, 31
negligence, 101, 139
Neisser, Albert, 129
Netherlands, 4, 75–86
Neumann, Robert, 38
neurosurgery, 152, 153
New World, 19
New York, 151
New Zealand, 139
Newsholme, Arthur, 131
newspapers, 34, 76, 77, 79, 80, 83–85,
    93, 151, 152, 159
notification. *See* compulsory
    notification
Nuremberg, 108

objections, 30, 34, 35, 37, 41, 115, 149,
    153, 154
objectivity, 42, 102, 154
onanism, 68
oral administration of drugs, 112, 113,
    115
oral sex, 63, 65
Oranienburg, 38
Ostertag, Berthold, 38
organ trade, 158
Osler, William, 1

pact with the Devil, 19
paediatric psychiatric hospital, 38
pain, 16, 64, 66, 137
Paré, 13
Paris, 31, 86
parliament, 40, 83
party politics, 92

pathological anatomy. *See* anatomy, pathological
Pathological Institute, 34, 35, 38
pathologists, 3, 30–32, 34–39, 41, 42, 151
pathology, 31, 32, 35, 39, 40, 42
  scientific, 30
patients, 2, 4, 5, 15, 31, 38, 40, 42, 62, 76–80, 82, 83, 96, 97, 99–101, 108–15, 117, 118, 120, 130, 132–35, 151, 155
  autonomy of, 121
  confidentiality of, 128, 140
  death of, 29, 31, 38, 153
  dissatisfied, 19
  experimental subjects, 119
  hospitalisation of, 112
  passive, 119
  relationship with practitioners, 6, 11, 19, 22, 29, 107, 108, 134, 150
  rights of, 29, 30, 107, 140
  treatment of, 81, 156
  views and feelings of, 83
pedagogy of fear, 18
penal code, 36, 92
penal consequences, 133
penal law, 38, 129
penal procedure, 15
penal regulations, 12, 129
penal servitude, 95
persecution, 2, 12, 19–22, 82
perverts, 55, 62, 63, 66, 68, 70
physicians, 3, 5, 11, 12–22, 29, 31, 34, 37–39, 42, 63, 76, 110, 113, 128, 134, 150, 152–57, 159, 160
Pichlmayr, Rudolf, 157
placebo, 81
Ploch, Marion, 159
pogroms, 18
poisonings, 13, 58
poisons, 138
police, 4, 14, 36, 62, 79, 91, 94–98, 100, 130, 136–39

Poller, Walter, 38
popularity, 75–86
Portocarrero, Cardinal, 21
Portugal, 18
postmortems, 3, 31, 34, 37, 41–43
practitioners, 4, 5, 19, 22, 29, 30, 75, 76, 109, 120. *See also* medical practitioners
  colonial, 119
  relationship with patients, 6, 11, 19, 22, 29, 107, 108, 134, 150
pregnancy, 15, 30, 98, 100, 101, 103, 136, 159
  tests, 99
  unwanted, 92, 93, 97, 103
prejudice, 32, 97, 115, 133
privilege, 14
professionalisation, 30, 40, 76
promiscuity, 136
propaganda, 119, 131, 132, 138
prosecutor, 97
Prosektor, 31
prostitution, 5, 68, 129, 130, 136, 139
Protestant Academy, Schleswig-Holstein, 154
Protestants, 3, 22, 75, 80, 82, 93, 153, 154
Prussia, 102, 128
  Ministry of Law, 35
  Ministry of Science, 34, 35, 39
psychiatry, 4, 38, 55, 58–62, 66, 67, 69
public health, 5, 80, 92, 96, 115, 127–33, 136–40
publicity, 4, 77, 79, 86
punishment, 12, 16, 59, 102
purity of blood, 14

quackery, 4, 19, 75, 76, 79–83, 86, 103
Quackery, Dutch Society for the Repression of, 75
Quackery, Monthly for the Repression of, 79, 80

Quackery, Society for the Repression of, 84–86
quinine, 111, 112

rabbi, 20
race, 5, 109, 120, 128, 130
regulations, 3, 13, 36, 40, 41, 42, 103, 131, 135, 136, 137. *See also* Defence of the Realm Regulations
  hospital, 34–36, 39
  legal, 2, 3, 12, 29, 30, 35, 37, 39, 42
  penal, 12, 129
  traditional, 36
Reichstag, 36, 130
relapses, 111–14, 116, 117
religious beliefs, 32, 33
religious leaders, 103
religious minorities, 18
religious orthodoxy, 15
reproduction, 66, 67, 92, 103
reputation, 15, 34, 67, 83, 99, 110
retribution, 91
revenge, 63, 96
revolution, 35, 150
rheumatism, 76, 77, 80, 83
Richardson, Ruth, 31
Ripper, Jack the, 62, 63
Ripper, Vacher the, 55–70
risk society, 150, 158
risks, 100, 115, 118, 120, 149, 150, 158
rivalry, 19
Roman Catholic Church. *See* Catholicism
Romantic medicine, 31
Roozendaal, 77, 78
Rorke, Margaret, 134
Ross, Ronald, 111
Rössle, Robert, 34, 36, 38, 39
Rotterdam, 78, 79, 82
Royal Commission, 131, 132

sacraments, 19

sadism, 4, 55–70
salary, 14, 22, 100
schistosomiasis, 115, 117
Schulte, Regina, 100
scientific medicine, 31–35, 40–42
Scotland, 83, 134–40
Scottish Royal Burghs, 137
Sequah, 75–86
Seville, 15, 20, 21
sexology, 55
sexuality, 55, 65, 98, 128, 137
sexually-transmitted diseases, 127–40
Shanghai, 38
Shumway, Norman E., 151
side effects, 109, 116, 117, 150, 158
Sierra Leone, 110, 115
simulation, 13
sleeping sickness, 110, 117, 118
social
  attitudes, 137, 150, 151
  behaviour, 97, 136
  changes, 70
  competency, 150
  conditions, 35
  consensus, 160
  constructs, 42
  control, 3, 5, 13, 22, 160
  costs, 158
  disgrace, 97
  ethics, 154
  forces, 4, 59
  harmony, 12
  history, 4, 7, 91, 92, 107, 128
  hygiene, 127, 133, 136, 138, 139
  influences, 59
  integration, 18
  intercourse, 136
  issues, 107
  legitimacy, 15, 22
  motives, 22
  order, 127
  patterns, 120
  phenomenon, 150
  power, 151
  practices, 12, 91

pressures, 4, 55
problems, 68
purity, 132, 135
respectability, 15, 22
risks, 158
status, 12–14, 21, 76
structures, 150, 158
theory, 150
values, 14
welfare, 41
workers, 97, 138
Social Democrats, 154, 157, 159
Social Insurance, 129, 130
Society for Combating VD, German,
129, 130
Society for Neurosurgery, German, 153
Society for the Prevention of Venereal
Diseases, 132
Society for the Repression of Quackery,
Dutch, 75
Society of Surgery, German, 153, 155
sodomy, 3, 22, 63, 67, 68
somnambules, 82
sorcery, 16
soul, 16
Spain, 2, 11–22, 155
Spanish Inquisition, 2, 11–22
spells, 19
STADA pharmaceutical company, 38
Stanford University, 151, 157
Stegeman, Peter, 82
Stephens, Professor John W.W., 111
stereotypes, 101, 102
stigmata, 60
Supreme Council, 14, 17
surgeons, 2, 3, 11, 12–22, 31, 149,
151–53, 157, 159
Sylvaticus, 13
symbolic actions, 85
synagogues, 20
syphilis, 69, 110, 128, 137

Tanganyika, 110, 117, 121

Tarde, Gabriel, 69
termination. *See* abortion
testimony, 97, 100, 101
theologians, 5, 16, 153–57, 159, 160
Thielecke, Helmut, 154
Third Reich, 38, 39
Tinde Laboratory, 117
tolerance, 4, 91
torture, 15
traditional beliefs, 32, 33, 39, 41, 42
traditionalism, 21
traditions, 22, 33, 34, 36, 37, 68, 92,
107, 108, 130, 133, 135–40, 150,
153
canonic, 13
civil, 13
intellectual, 15
legal, 13
transplantation, 30, 149, 151–59
treatment, 77–81, 83, 107, 113–17, 129,
132, 140, 156
alternative, 81
baseline clinical data for, 114
centres, 131, 132
compulsory, 128, 130, 131, 133, 134,
139
courses of, 109, 115, 136
discontinued, 132–35
experimental, 117
facilities, 134
mass, 115
medical, 108
modes of, 112
neglect of, 128, 131
of malaria, 111, 113
of sleeping sickness, 118
of venereal disease, 131, 134, 135
process, 114, 138
refusal of, 114, 135
regimes, 112, 113, 130
schedules, 111
strategies, 135
v. punishment, 59
Trevethin, Lord, 134

trials, 12, 13, 16–22, 38, 39, 55, 58, 59, 61, 67, 91–103
  clinical, 108, 114, 117, 120
  Nuremburg, 108
tropical diseases, 109, 110
tropical medicine, 110, 111, 117, 120. *See also* Liverpool School of Tropical Medicine
*Trypanosoma rhodesiense*, 117, 118
trypanosomiasis, 110, 117, 119
Tryparsamide, 117
Tübingen, 38
  Institute of Brain Research, 38

*unbefugter übergriff*, 37
United Brethren in Christ Mission, 115, 116
United Free Church, 138
United States of America. *See* America
universities, 15, 22, 32
University Clinic, Königsberg, 37
university education, 12, 19, 75
University Hospital, Erlangen, 159
University of
  Freiburg, 30, 40, 43
  Giessen, 41
  Hamburg, 152, 154
  Munich, 155
  Stanford, 151, 157

Vacher, Joseph, 55–70
Valencia, 15
Valladolid, 15
venereal disease, 5, 127–40
venereologists, 129, 130, 132, 138
Venlo, 81, 84
Virchow, Rudolf, 32, 35, 40
  Chair of Pathology, 35
  Rudolf Virchow Hospital, Berlin, 38
  Rudolf Virchow Institute, Berlin, 40
voluntarism, 132, 134, 135, 138–40
volunteers, 113, 114, 117, 118, 119
*vorzugsweises Aneignungsrecht*, 37

voyeurism, 55, 60

War
  First World, 40, 92, 110–14, 121, 129, 132, 139
  Napoleonic, 128
  Second World, 121, 134–36, 138
  Spanish Succession, 20
War Cabinet, 132, 136
War Office, 111, 114
war pathology, 40
Ward, D.C.L., 134
Washkansky, Louis, 151–53
Weimar Republic, 3, 41, 42, 91–103, 139
welfare, 41, 92, 121, 130, 136, 138, 139
widows, 20, 34
wise-women, 96
witchcraft, 16, 19, 119
Wolferstan, Harold, 110
women
  attitudes of, 93
  beliefs of, 95
  emancipation of, 92
  role of, 4, 97
Women, National Council of, 139
Women's Citizens Association, 139
women's movement, 128, 129, 132, 139
women's organisations, 135, 139
women's rights, 92
working class, 95, 96, 99, 100, 103, 136

Yorke, Warrington, 110, 115

Zacchia, Paolo, 13
Zapata, Diego Mateo, 21
Zaragoza, 15
*Zeitung, Berliner*, 34
*Zeitung, Frankfurter Allgemeine*, 152
Zemon Davies, Natalie, 95
Zenker, Rudolf, 153, 155, 156
Zola, 62